Losing Us

A DEMENTIA CAREGIVER'S JOURNEY

ROSELLA M. LESLIE

FriesenPress

One Printers Way
Altona, MB R0G 0B0
Canada

www.friesenpress.com

Published by
QUINTESSENTIAL PUBLISHING GROUP

Cover Design: Corinna Enevoldson
Cover Photo: Lori Alvarez

BRITISH COLUMBIA ARTS COUNCIL | BRITISH COLUMBIA

Supported by the Province of British Columbia

The author acknowledges and is grateful for the financial support of the B.C.
Arts Council through their Project Assistance for Creative Writers grant
program.

ISBN
978-1-03-915641-8 (Hardcover)
978-1-03-915640-1 (Paperback)
978-1-03-915642-5 (eBook)

1. BIOGRAPHY & AUTOBIOGRAPHY, PERSONAL MEMOIRS

Distributed to the trade by The Ingram Book Company

This book is dedicated to all caregivers and to the many kind and caring people who helped me on my journey.

Table of Contents

Introduction

My goal in adding yet another book about dementia to the bookshelves of the world is not just to tell the story of my journey as a caregiver or of my husband's slow transformation from lover, confidant, and best friend to a stranger whom I sometimes wasn't even sure I liked. Telling that story as recorded in the daily journal I kept and sharing the poems I wrote along the way certainly played a role in my decision to write the book, but neither drove me to relive a journey that most people would happily leave behind.

In truth, the force that motivated me throughout the writing of *Losing Us* was multifaceted. First, I believe that in sharing my story and the insights and strategies I learned as the journey progressed, I can help others to be the best caregivers they can be without sacrificing their health, future, or sense of self. Second, my experiences might help them avoid some of the pitfalls that I encountered—such as believing that looking after someone with dementia is a one-person job, when, in fact, it requires a whole army of workers to provide the greatest amount of comfort and care to the person with dementia while decreasing the physical, mental, and emotional stress of the primary caregiver.

Third, and almost as important, I wanted my story to inform the community, to allow others to understand what help the caregiver needs, why they need it and how that help can best be delivered. And by community, I don't mean just family and friends. I mean local organizations such as community services, seniors' centres, churches, and federal, provincial, and local government agencies.

In writing this book I have exposed many of the negative emotions and cruelties that I was guilty of during this journey. They are not feelings or actions I am proud of, but they are very human reactions to the grief, frustration, and exhaustion that, despite their best intentions, overtake caregivers, often on a daily basis, especially when the person being cared for enters the later stages of dementia. I share these incidents to reassure new caregivers that they have not become monsters if they find themselves reacting in a similar manner but instead are receiving cries for help from their inner selves because they are reaching the limits of their endurance. And I point out that one caregiver's limits cannot be compared to those of another, because each of us is an individual with unique stores of strengths and weaknesses. Paying attention to that inner cry for help and reaching out to their community is what will enable them to survive this journey and have a future they can enjoy when the journey is over.

I have not even a fragment of regret for the twelve years I spent as my husband's primary caregiver. I did the best that I could, and even during angry, soul-crushing moments I discovered to my surprise that I was strong and resilient. My knowledge of the human brain expanded as I dealt with the dips and circles and switches in logic and mood that can occur as dementia progresses. Most of all, my life was enriched by the kindness and support of my family and friends and the people in both the dementia care-giving community and the larger community beyond.

There is much yet to be learned about this disease, and many more resources are vitally needed to support caregivers, but I have faith that the generosity that exists in our communities and the dedication of those involved in dementia care will eventually result in a world in which looking after a person with dementia is not a prison sentence but a treasured gift.

I truly hope that *Losing Us* will help to create that world.

CHAPTER ONE

Present

TAKE OFF

There is a moment
On an airplane
That comes
After the doors are sealed,
Seat belts are fastened,
The runway is reached,
The engines rev,
And the pavement slides past
The windows
Faster and faster
Until the wheels lift,
The sky is breached
And there is no going back.
It is that moment
When all control
Has slipped from my grasp
That I let go
And allow what will happen
To happen.

I need to fly
More often.

Young love is a world unto itself. A world where nothing matters except the bond that has magically formed between two individuals. Where each day starts with the touch of a hand, the warmth of a body pressed close, the tender expression on the face and in the eyes, and the softly whispered, "I love you," that spreads warmth through one's whole being. This is not a world reserved only for the young, but I would have scoffed had someone suggested seven months ago that it could be otherwise. Certainly, it was not a world I ever considered entering again, especially not after seventy-two years of living, the last twelve of them devoted to caregiving, and the past five of those caregiving years spent watching my love and life partner, John, slip further and further away from me as dementia destroyed more and more of his brain. And yet, there I was, head-over-heels in love with Brian. He had been equally certain that the time for romance was long past, having travelled roughly the same journey through dementia caregiving as I had and was as stunned as I to find new love.

We were lost in the wonderment of it all one soft spring evening as we held hands across a table at a waterside restaurant and so immersed in whispering "I love you," that we didn't see the rather exuberant lady, appropriately masked for COVID protection, approaching our table.

"Pardon me," she exclaimed loudly, "but I just have to know! How long have you two been together?"

She was beaming not at the two eighteen-year-olds who had taken up residence in our bodies, but at an old couple who were obviously still very much in love. Not wanting to burst her bubble of delight, we fumbled for a simple, yet truthful, explanation.

"We aren't married," I sputtered. "My husband has dementia . . . he's in care . . ."

"We've been together seven months," said Brian. "My wife had the same thing."

"My husband doesn't know me," I added, desperate for understanding.

The woman stared at us for a faint second then exclaimed, "Well, good on you! You just keep grabbing that happiness. It's wonderful to see!"

As she bounced off to another area of the restaurant, Brian and I squeezed each other's hands.

"We really have to come up with a short answer," I said, and we both chuckled.

But there was no short answer. The circumstances that had brought us to this moment were complicated, heartbreaking, and almost soul-destroying. They weren't single, isolated incidents but years of struggling. Nor could we explain in a few social seconds how it was that, after years of inching through a long, dark tunnel of despair, our paths had wobbled together, and we found ourselves awash in the light of hope and possibilities.

To understand, one would have to go back to the very beginning.

HOT TUB ON A FROSTY NIGHT

Floating easily in a watery womb,
Warmth and wonder coalescing,
Frost in the air and a million stars
Twinkling in the dark midnight sky
While the snow-white moon
Drapes shadowed treetops with light.

I am whole in this place,
All parts of me gathered in one
Delicious package of content;
No past nor future, only a now
And a quiet soul absorbed
By the splendor of this night.

CHAPTER TWO

The Diagnosis

IN THE BEGINNING

I didn't want it to be so,
Kept denying what my eyes
And every sense within me
Were observing.

He was too tired to pay attention,
The road too wet to stop for the light,
The room so noisy when I spoke,
He could not hear.

I fought the burden that I sensed
Was heading my way, insisting
I would not give up my life
To nurture his.

Until the verdict was rendered
And I was forced to accept
Abandoning him was not
The choice for me.

In the fall of 2009 my husband, John, was diagnosed with vascular dementia. He had just celebrated his eighty-first birthday, and I would be sixty-one before the year was out.

At that time my knowledge of dementia was limited. John had told me how his Grandma Annie had been placed in a care home for her own safety. She had been living with his mother, Isabel, on the outskirts of Portland and had a habit of disappearing—one time turning up at a house near the downtown area where she'd lived as a girl. But John was always bothered by the fact that Annie had nothing to do in the care home. "She liked to knit," he told me. "They should give her some wool and some knitting needles." (Today I can understand why that never happened.) Once when he visited her in the home, she asked him to hold out his hands. When he did so, she spat in one of them. "Make a wish in the other," she said, "and what do you have the most of?" Until the day she died, Isabel never stopped feeling guilty for giving up on caring for her mother.

I remembered, too, visiting an aunt who was in the later stages of dementia. She could not grasp who I was, and I couldn't understand a word she said. A few years after that visit, John and I went to see my uncle in a home for people with dementia. He wanted our help to get himself out of there, and I was almost swayed until he pointed out a field beyond the home where gigantic jack rabbits lived.

"The person with dementia does not *suffer* from dementia," a doctor once told me, and this is generally true. But sometimes the diagnosis is made early enough that the victim is still able to understand the diagnosis and the prognosis. Each person with dementia presents with a unique personality, physical, and mental abilities. In the same way each caregiver's life history, genetic makeup, mental and physical health issues affect their ability to cope with the anxiety and frustration of caring for someone with dementia while dealing at the same time with the ongoing demands of their own lives. Added to this mix is the prior relationship shared by the caregiver and the dementia victim, which can include old angers, resentments, and betrayals.

I had no past issues with John, but I did have a chronic anxiety disorder and was ill-equipped to handle the stress of caregiving, especially when combined with developing my literary career and taking care of extended family problems and social obligations. Even our good, strong marriage wasn't perfect.

John and I had met in late 1980 at Clowhom Falls, BC, a wilderness area forty kilometres by boat from the village of Sechelt, which is a small community squeezed between the Inland Sea—comprised of Sechelt, Salmon, and Narrows inlets—and the Strait of Georgia. At the time, he was a divorced landed immigrant with four grown children and six grandchildren—all living in the United States—and the caretaker and guide for a private fishing lodge. I, as a wannabe-writer, had taken up residence in a float house one bay down the inlet. He offered me a job at the lodge, and I gradually began spending more time on his side of the inlet than my own. We were married in 1984 and our son, Nathan, was born two years later.

Perhaps the greatest issue affecting our marriage was John's impaired hearing. He was already growing deaf when we met, and eventually even hearing aids were not helping him. It was partly for this reason (and partly so that Nathan could attend school) that he retired from his dream job at Clowhom Falls, and we moved to Sechelt where we had purchased a four-acre property not far from our beloved inlets.

By 1994 writing notes was my only means of communicating with John. This method failed miserably at times, such as when we were arguing as he was driving us down the freeway. It is hard to yell at someone in print, especially when they can't take their eyes off the road. Needless to say, he won most of the arguments, while I stewed in frustration in the passenger seat. Then, in the fall of 1997, John was approved for a cochlear implant and admitted to St. Paul's Hospital where his right cochlea was removed and twenty-four electrodes that fit on a disk about the size of a dime were implanted in its place. After a six-week recovery period, a speech processor was connected and John's audiologist, Dr. Sipke Pijl, tuned each electrode to accept a different frequency.

"It was amazing," the doctor told me. "Most people reject the high notes because they are too uncomfortable, but John embraced them. He said it had been so long since he'd heard them that he didn't want to miss them." It was a miracle-moment when the tuning was completed, and John heard our son's voice for the first time in years.

Although we were now able to communicate better than we ever had, unless John was paying attention, he would not realize that I was speaking, even if I was standing right beside him. Thus, I often had to repeat what I had said. Nor was he averse to using this technology to his advantage. More than once, after having his say in an argument, he would turn the processor off so he did not have to listen to my rebuttal, and I cannot count the number of times he would call out a question from upstairs, knowing full well he would not hear my response unless I was in the same room. It never occurred to him to walk to where I was—he just kept calling out the question until I came to him.

Another of his peculiarities was to leave the last part of whatever job he was tackling undone. A few blocks of wood not chopped. The final piece of siding never put in place. Grapes carefully tended but not harvested. For years I blamed this on butterflies—thoughts that would flutter into his brain and divert him from his original goal, sometimes bringing him back to the starting point . . . and sometimes not.

But these were minor irritants that I had learned to live with, just as he had learned to live with my own foibles, and overall, our marriage was solid. John fished and hunted, raised bantam chickens, and grew grapes and apples. I looked after the house and financial matters and pursued my writing career. We were both actively involved in the community, he with our local ratepayers' association and helping at the Sunshine Coast Salmonid Enhancement

Society's hatchery, and me with the Festival of the Written Arts, parent advisory councils, and other school-based organizations.

It was because of the busy lives we were leading and John's impaired hearing that it took me a while to notice that he was also having cognitive difficulties. He would forget things I'd told him only an hour earlier or not remember where he had left this tool or that. Or he would fail to recognize someone we'd known forever. It didn't help that these changes occurred when we were already coping with serious upheavals in our lives. To augment our limited income, I was providing day care for my young niece and, while still doing this, had started a bed and breakfast. My father passed away and only a year later I helped nurse my mother through the final stages of terminal lung cancer that had metastasized to her bones and lymph glands. Within the next decade one of my brothers died, our son graduated from high school and left home, John's mother died, and his son by his previous marriage fought and won a long battle with leukemia. Within such turmoil who wouldn't forget a few things?

But John's cognitive failures were not consistent. He would be fine for a few weeks or months and then suddenly do something strange, such as walking out of a store where we were shopping together without telling me that he was leaving. After searching the store several times and steaming with anger, I would find him sitting happily in the car. "I couldn't see you," he'd say calmly when I finished ranting, as if I was the one at fault for not understanding that leaving was the most sensible thing for him to do. After all, how could he tell me he was leaving if he couldn't find me?

Like many good fishermen and hunters, John liked to exaggerate stories of his catches, and I had always accepted this as part of his persona until his exaggerations began to impact our relationships with friends and neighbours. He accused them of stealing tools that he had misplaced or fabricated elaborate stories, such as one about a local business dumping toxic waste into the ocean.

When, in private, I confronted him about the accuracy of his statements, he became angry and defensive and so passionate about his rightness that I'd walk away certain that I was wrong.

One day while Googling some of the abnormalities I was noticing in John's behaviour, I found myself at an online screening test for dementia. Today organizations such as the Alzheimer Society of BC discourage such tests because they often give a false positive, but I was desperate for answers and so, without letting him know their purpose, I asked John the questions on the test and entered his answers. The positive result so frightened me that I deleted the site from my computer's history.

Unfortunately, that did not stop John's memory lapses or his increasingly bizarre stories, and I found myself thinking more and more about the claim on one Googled site that an underlying, treatable medical condition—such as anaemia or depression—might cause dementia-like symptoms. A visit to our family physician was recommended, but I hesitated, worried that by sharing my suspicions, I would prejudice the doctor so he would no longer see John as a vital, intelligent man. I was also haunted by "what-ifs" such as: What if the doctor came up with the diagnosis I feared, and he recommended that his driver's licence be cancelled? What if friends and family found out and as a result stopped taking him seriously?

It was all so worrisome that I put the doctor's number away and went back to making excuses for John's behaviour, downplaying his accusations that a neighbour had borrowed this or that without returning it, or his insistence that I had hidden the wallet he couldn't find. It was harder to accept the questions he repeated over and over even after I had given and made sure he had heard and understood my answers. Strangely, as if he, too, sensed something was wrong, he was suddenly afraid to walk in certain areas or to go out in the boat when the weather was unpredictable. And somewhere along the line, he stopped being a co-leader in our marriage and began deferring to me to make decisions.

In the end it was a radio documentary that claimed there were medications available to slow down the symptoms of dementia that prompted me to make an appointment with the doctor. John resisted. Save for those rare moments when he was aware of his confusion, he didn't think he had a problem. He had an explanation for every fear, forgotten memory, and lapse in judgement—the weather was unstable, or I had spoken too softly for him to hear my plans or instructions, or there was too much noise or confusion for him to think straight. But I persisted and finally, to please me, he agreed to go for a checkup, though only if I went with him.

The doctor didn't seem surprised by my concerns about John's mental abilities. As if it was an everyday issue, he carried out a physical exam, ordered some laboratory tests, and had John complete a Mini-Mental State Exam (MMSE). The results seemed to surprise the doctor, and after administering a different test just to be sure, he told us somewhat reluctantly that John had mild cognitive impairment and that this would eventually lead to dementia.

The diagnosis confirmed my suspicions and was certainly better than a diagnosis of full-blown dementia, but I felt as if my whole world had suddenly come to a crashing stop.

"How long?" I managed to ask. My mouth was so dry the words came out garbled.

The look the doctor gave me was kind. "There is no way of knowing. It could be months or years." He hesitated then said, "There is evidence that in some cases the progression can be slowed down with a drug called Donepezil HCL. If you want, we can try it out."

I nodded, and as I gathered our coats and prepared to leave, he wrote out the prescription and handed it to me. "There is support available," he said gently. "You won't be alone in this."

Rosella M. Leslie

I managed to hold back my tears long enough to thank him before stumbling out of the office. John followed, completely oblivious to the meaning of the doctor's diagnosis, having heard only the word "mild," and as we left the clinic, he cheerfully suggested we stop for a coffee and a treat. Although I desperately wanted to go home where I could hide in our bedroom, bury my head in a pillow, and cry my heart out, I managed a wobbly smile and said, as he had said a million times to me, "Yes, dear."

12

IT BEGINS

It begins with a lost word that is never found,
Keys that mysteriously vanish,
A familiar place not recognized,
A red light not seen . . . or ignored,
The neglecting of a task that used to be easy
But now furrows the brow with frustration,
The same story told and retold not in days
But within the hour and sometimes the minute,
Or the unrelenting questions asked and re-asked
No matter how many times the answer is given.

It begins with a strange behaviour that is dismissed
As a momentary blip that everyone experiences—
Until the blips are too numerous to ignore
And doubts creep in, spawning internal arguments:
Are the missing objects and forgotten tasks
Simply a result of aging or something more sinister?
Is the confusion just joking around as claimed
Or a symptom that should not be ignored?
Can these anomalies be exposed without destroying
The dignity of the one who is loved and cherished?

It begins with an insistence that the signs are wrong;
With so wanting to believe that the mind is whole
That accusations of not trying hard enough are uttered
And fabrications corrected as if they are deliberate;
With a growing sense that the pilot is leaving the plane
In the hands of an untrained and unwilling passenger;
With tears and fears and the D-word not spoken aloud
Lest it turn suspicion into irretrievable reality;
It begins with an acceptance that failure to ask the question
Will not change the answer.

It begins.

It begins.

CHAPTER THREE

Mindfulness

A SINGLE STEP

A single step. That's all it takes.
One foot stretched forward
And planted firm . . . and somehow
The second foot follows.
The trick is, don't look ahead—
Therein lies exhaustion and defeat.
Instead, focus on the moment—
The ground beneath your feet,
A single bramble that needs cutting,
A weed that needs pulling,
A stick of wood that needs carrying.
No plans. No expectations.
No threat of failure.
Just one step forward and then another;
One minute of endurance, and then two,
Until the wait is over, the discomfort eased.
One step at a time. It is all we really have.
Anything else is fantasy.

There is a fine line between sorrow and joy. Sometimes, for me, that line is almost tangible, and I feel as if I can choose on which side of it I will stand. On one side is an angry railing against the situation I'm in—a sad desperation filled with dark thoughts of the husband I've lost and a mountain of things I've said or done wrong or haven't said or done at all. The other side is filled with love and laughter and gratitude for the good that still exists in the world. Here there is an acceptance that I did not cause John's dementia and cannot cure or control it, and a realization that there is no right or wrong behaviour, only endless opportunities to do my best and, when that is not enough, to collect my resources and try again.

When I am running or hiking, especially through the woods where mindfulness is almost automatic, it is easier to hang out on the good side. Although one of my brothers hates the term "mindfulness" as he thinks it is trendy and meaningless, I see it more as a mind *full* of what I choose to put into it. It gets so full that it pushes out the stuff I don't want (at least for the duration of the exercise) and gives me a chance to rebuild my mental and emotional—and consequently my physical—strengths.

Running requires a certain kind of concentration, partly to manage the path, watching out for dips or obstacles that could cause me to trip or twist an ankle and land face-first in the dirt, and partly to keep going. It is a great way to discharge pent-up angers and frustrations. My whole focus becomes centred on the rhythm of my feet pounding on the path, the movement of my legs, the regulation of my breathing, and the steady thumping of my heart. When dark thoughts threaten to invade this space, I count—one-step, two-step, three-step—all the way to one hundred then start again. By the time the run is over, my body is flooded with endorphins and the euphoric sense that I am strong enough to conquer all obstacles.

Hiking in the woods is truly mindful, engaging all my senses. I breathe deeply, inhaling air tinged—depending on the season— with frost or warm breezes and the scents of moss and earth, sweet vapours rising from pine needles warming in the summer sun or in the fall the musty-sweet aroma of maple leaves drying on the ground. My eyes probe the vegetation along the trail, the green and gold shades of mosses, ferns that start out as tiny, hairy curls and gradually unfold to majestic branches, the deep, thick crevices in the bark of an aged fir tree, the multi-textured fungi shaped like interplanetary creatures clinging to decaying logs or hugging the trunks of dead or dying trees that are pock-marked with wood-pecker holes meticulously carved into identical shapes to become ideal hiding places for all manner of wildlife. All the while, I am alert to the sounds of the forest—the eerie squeal of two trees rubbing against each other, the warning *kuk kuk kuk* from a squir-rel on a branch above the trail, the high-pitched scream of an unseen eagle, the cheerful song of a robin, the trill of a blackbird, or the soft *clump clump* of my footsteps. When I feel hungry, I pull a bit of licorice fern root from the trunk of a maple tree, carefully peel away the outer coating, and chew the woody root, filling my mouth with its bitter-sweet flavour. In season I enjoy a feast of berries—juicy salmon berries, tangy red huckleberries, mellowly sweet thimbleberries, and, if I'm lucky and arrive before the bears have cleaned them out, the delicately sweet flavour of wild straw-berries. All the while, my cheeks are soothed by the breeze created by my walking, and my legs feel strong as they swing and lift and lower. Sometimes I pause and run my fingers along the bark of a rugged fir or sinewed cedar, and occasionally tease myself by touching the tip of a berry vine thorn. Always I end up feeling intensely alive as the phytoncides emitted by the trees and plants around wash away my cares and rebuild my immune system.

This may sound poetic and fanciful, perhaps even a little sappy (forgive the tree pun), but runs and hikes are some of the primary things that have sustained me throughout my journey as a care-giver. If nothing else, they are a reminder that there is more to life than dementia and that, when all the caring and stress and hurting is over, the world will still be there waiting for me to embrace it. Nor is it limited to hikes or runs. I have experienced the same release, the same equilibrium, paddling a kayak on a calm sea or walking along the shore, picking up shells and bits of driftwood or beach glass and allowing my mind to explore very real possibilities—books I'm going to write, trips I'm going to take, community work I'm going to do. Dreams and plans that will still be waiting when the time is right.

LETTING GO

Today I let go of expectations,
Just let myself be,
Felt the summer sun on my face,
Saw a light in someone's eyes,
Searched for mushrooms in the woods.
I wasn't giddy with laughter
Or overjoyed or excited,
But I was at peace—
Just me and the world kicking back.
Funny thing was, by letting go,
By not trying,
I was kinder to you
And when you carried in wood
That was meant to dry for another year,
I did not grit my teeth or snarl.
Instead, I smiled and thought,
Tomorrow I will put it back,
But for today, I will just let it be.

CHAPTER FOUR

Denial

LUMOSITY EXERCISES

You sit beside me
Focussed on the screen,
Clicking on numbered frogs
Or coloured squares
Or patterned blocks,
Determined to defeat
This vile disease
Invading your brain.

As your guide, I watch
And patiently wait
To advance the program,
Praising your score
Explaining rules
For the next game
Then giving you
The chance to succeed.

It doesn't hurt you,
And I tell myself
It's bringing us closer.
Sometimes we laugh;
Sometimes I cry,
Watching you try,
Hoping this isn't
As good as it gets.

If I was the rational person that I've always thought myself to be, my next move after receiving the diagnosis of John's dementia would have been to put supports in place, inform family and friends, and get our affairs in order. But the way I saw it, once people heard about John's dementia, they would stop seeing him as an intelligent man and start treating him as they might a child, dismissing anything he might say or do as nonsense. So instead of reaching out for help or putting things in order, I told no one and made no outward changes. *We will try the Donepezil first*, I told myself, *before making any radical shifts to our lives.*

Caregiver opinions on the benefits of Donepezil HCL are mixed. Some say it really helped, others say it made no difference. Unfortunately for John, its effects were devastating. Over the six months of taking the medication he experienced headaches, muscle aches, and terrible dreams. One day, he mixed up his mother with his grandmother when remembering a past story. But the worst of his reactions was a depression that often had him in tears. To combat this, we stopped watching the news, and I refrained from sharing any negative family issues. By April his doctor agreed that the medication was not working and discontinued his prescription. Within a week John was feeling better, and although his short-term memory issues were still present, we resigned ourselves to letting nature take its course.

Almost.

Even before John's diagnosis I had enrolled him in Lumosity, an online program that was advertised as a means to train the brain and improve cognitive abilities. Since he had never used a computer, we had been doing the exercises together, with me typing in his responses to the questions or problems presented. Now I expanded our exercise time to include some of the tasks he had been asked to do on the MMSE test—remembering words, drawing a clock, and inserting the correct time and drawing a cube. I also introduced an exercise regime of walking every day and added vitamins B, D, and folic acid supplements to his daily diet. Gradually his cognitive abilities increased, and that fall I breathed a sigh of relief when he passed his medical for the renewal of his driver's licence. I credited the improvement to the physical exercises, the supplements, and the Lumosity exercises.

This cognitive improvement did not last forever, but over the next few years, John's decline was so insignificant that I began to believe that our strategy had reversed or at least halted the damage that had been done to his brain. He continued to fish, trailering his boat to and from the water and successfully launching it, often under conditions that would cause other boaters to give up. Occasionally he drove by himself to Vancouver Island to fish with a friend at Brown's Bay. Soon I was focussing less on him and more on my writing. I attended literary events and went on book tours, leaving John at home by himself. In late 2011, as he did every fall, John pulled my friend's boat from the water and trailered it to her place. Scorning our help, he insisted on securing the boat to the trailer using ropes and at least one hundred perfectly tied fisherman's knots. As I watched him back the trailer up my friend's steep, curving driveway and park the boat exactly where she wanted it, I was more convinced than ever that his memory lapses were nothing more than normal aging.

Sechelt and the rest of the Sunshine Coast, is part of the Lower Mainland, and not an island as some folks suppose, but because of the mountainous terrain to the east, the only access to it is by ferries. A terminal at Earl's Cove on the north end of the Sechelt Peninsula provides a link to Saltery Bay and Powell River, while another terminal at Langdale, twenty-six kilometres south of Sechelt, connects Langdale with Horseshoe Bay and Vancouver. Sailing time for this latter route is normally forty minutes. Although this ferry system is inconvenient for many travellers, it does mean that our local roads don't have a high traffic volume, making driving much easier, and it is often a shock when we encounter the speed and noise of city streets.

For someone with dementia, this shift is also confusing, and as a result, over time John grew increasingly anxious when driving in the city. After one rainy night when he drove over a cement curb leading onto the Stanley Park Causeway in Vancouver, I insisted that I would do our city driving from now on, and except for his occasional trips to Brown's Bay, his driving would be limited to our own small community. While I was confident that he could do this safely and responsibly, the Department of Motor Vehicles had other ideas. After his eighty-fourth birthday in 2012, John was required to report to the DriveAble testing office. To keep his driver's licence, he had to take a road test in a DriveAble vehicle, which had an automatic transmission. John, who was used to the standard transmission in his truck, could not adapt to the change. Consequently, he failed the driving test and the computer test that followed and was instructed to surrender his driver's licence.

Convinced that it was the unfamiliar vehicle and his lack of computer skills that had caused him to fail, I officially protested the cancellation of his licence, and in due course he was given the opportunity to retest. By then I had worked with him on the computer, teaching him to enter his own responses for the Lumosity exercises and practising the driver's tests available on the ICBC website. When the day came for his new DriveAble test, he was able to do the exercises, and when he could not hear the multiple-choice options he was given, he was able to let the tester know so they could be written down for him. As a result, he passed that test and a road test that was administered in his own truck, and his driver's licence was restored.

That October John was due for his next MMSE exam. As they chitchatted before the test, John showed the doctor his speech processor and explained in detail how it worked.

"Anyone who can manage that system is not suffering from dementia," said the doctor and put the test away.

As the next years crept by, John and I continued with our lives as normal. Or so it seemed. Looking back on it now, I realize that our definition of "normal" was constantly shifting, but it was so gradual that I didn't notice it was happening. I had become used to John being paranoid about people stealing his things, and it didn't seem to be a big deal when this expanded to hiding things such as his wallet before retiring at night and then forgetting not just where he'd placed the wallet but that he'd done anything with it at all. "Someone took it," he'd say. He could never come up with the name of who that "someone" might be, but he was beginning to look very carefully at me.

Nor did I realize until much later that he was avoiding fishing by himself, even in the best of weather, or that his trips on the water were becoming limited to days when I could go with him or when he could go with a friend or family member. One day while we were fishing, we stopped, as we often did, to collect oysters, and as was his custom, John let me off on the rocks then moved the boat offshore to await my signal that I had filled my bucket with oysters. It occurred to me as I was trying to attract his attention that being left on the rocks by someone with short term memory issues might not be the safest thing to do. (He never did forget me there, but the idea resulted in a published short story, "Stuck on a Rock.")

There was also a day when John disappeared. His habit of returning to the car when we were shopping without letting me know he was leaving had persisted, and no matter how many times I told him I would not leave without him, he'd forget and do it again. On this occasion, while babysitting our granddaughter in Vancouver's West End, we took her to a pharmacy to purchase diapers. Stressing that we needed to stay together, I parked our granddaughter's stroller close to me while I studied the row of diapers for sale, trying to decide which brand and size to buy, and it wasn't until I'd made my choice that I discovered John was no longer with us. I immediately searched inside the store, and when I couldn't find him, I went through the checkout, stuffed the diapers into the stroller basket, and hurried outside to the busy street.

Cars zoomed past, buses stopped to discharge and take on passengers, and an endless stream of people paraded past in each direction, but John was nowhere to be seen. Pushing the stroller and praying that granddaughter would not start to fuss, I returned to the store and went up and down every aisle so many times that the security guard stopped me. I explained my problem and he, too, began to search, but John was not there.

Growing increasingly desperate, I called our son who was working at a store in a different part of the West End, and after I'd reassured him that it was his father and not his daughter who was lost, he said he had not seen his dad, but promised to keep an eye out for him. John had no key to our son's apartment building, but not knowing what else to do, I walked back there. When he wasn't waiting outside as I'd hoped, my imagination went wild. I envisioned him boarding a bus, intending to go back to the ferry but was instead being discharged in a less-than-safe part of the city. Growing frantic, I made two more trips back and forth to the drug store and was close to tears when our son finally called to say that John had just arrived at the store. I will never know how he managed to navigate the streets to find his way there, and I was too relieved to do anything but hug him when we got back together. Still, a warning bell clanged in my head. *This is not simply aging, and it definitely isn't normal.*

In the months that followed I began to pay closer attention to the things that kept disappearing from our home such as garden clippers, screw drivers and keys, especially the keys to the pad-locks that John insisted we use to secure sheds, boat trailers, lawnmowers, and anything else he could fasten one onto. After cutting several of these locks with a hacksaw, I finally invested in an electric angle grinder and soon became an expert in its use.

In the fall of 2014 we celebrated John's eighty-sixth birthday. It was a smaller gathering than in years previous because many of his fishing companions, including his friend at Brown's Bay, had died, and others had moved away. That December we made a bus trip to the city, and while keeping a close eye on John so he did not wander, I spent a delightful day looking after our granddaughter. By late afternoon, however, we were both exhausted, and because John walked very slowly, we left early to catch the only bus that would connect us with the 5:30 ferry home. Since the next sailing wouldn't leave until 7:30, I panicked when, still half a block away, I saw the bus arrive at our stop.

"You walk," I said hastily to John, "and I'll run ahead and ask the driver to wait." Without waiting to see if John had heard me, I sprinted for the bus. The driver kindly kept the door open, and I swung about expecting to find John coming slowly behind me. Instead, he was sprawled on the sidewalk, his eyeglasses shattered, and blood trickling down his face from a wound in his forehead. He was dazed and clearly could not understand what was happening as I helped him to sit up, aided by several kind bystanders. Moments later, emergency vehicles arrived and after a temporary bandage was placed on the wound, he was loaded into an ambulance. Riding in the cab of the ambulance as we sped towards the hospital, I had a hard time holding back tears of fear, shame, and guilt, blaming myself for putting the goal of catching that damned bus ahead of my husband's welfare.

Fortunately, John's injuries were minor. His forehead was stitched, and my sister and her husband volunteered to drive us to the ferry, but the incident forced me to take a hard look at just how far John's cognitive impairment had progressed. I began to take stock of the many signs I'd been dismissing as aging—not just his hiding things or repeating the same question again and again but also the slowness with which he did everything and how unsteady his gait had become. It was time, I realized, to visit a lawyer to make arrangements for handling John's legal and financial affairs while he was still deemed capable of making decisions for himself.

In February we both signed documents giving each other power of attorney and representation agreements with enhanced authority for health and personal care—including Do Not Resuscitate (DNR) orders. When I explained to John that the DNR order would be used if he were ever admitted to a long-term care facility, he said emphatically, "I don't want to go to a nursing home!"

"And I don't want you to," I said gently, "but there may be a time in the future when I can't care for you anymore."

"Then hit me over the head with a frying pan," he said.

It took a while to convince him that I was never going to do that, but eventually he did sign, as I had signed, the documents that would not prolong our lives for longer than was absolutely necessary should permanent long-term care ever be required.

At the same time, as we were getting our legal affairs in order, I had one of our two bathrooms—both located downstairs—enlarged to include a walk-in shower and handrails in preparation for a day when John might need help with bathing. My goal, as always, was to keep him at home until the end of this journey, something I was sure I could manage with proper planning.

That spring, prompted by an ad in the local paper, I registered for a workshop on dementia sponsored by the Alzheimer Society of British Columbia. *I don't really need to be here,* I told myself as I listened to the instructor and the caregivers of people who had far more advanced dementia than John was exhibiting. But by the time the workshop was over, I had learned enough about dementia to accept the fact that John was not ever going to recover the memories he'd lost nor the ability to manage his life without help.

That night I emailed our son in Vancouver and John's son and three daughters in the United States and warned them that, if they wanted to see their father while he still knew who they were and could interact with them, this was the time to schedule a visit.

A few months later a dear friend who was like a third son to John and called him Pops invited us on a three-day visit in his cabin cruiser to Princess Louisa Inlet. John eagerly agreed and he did well on the trip. Although he'd been there before, he was enthralled by Chatterbox Falls at the end of the inlet and the mountains surrounding it and was even able to cast a line into Queen's Inlet. On the way home, however, he grew increasingly disoriented, mistaking boulders on deserted beaches for houses and believing the entrance to the Skookumchuck Rapids was the Columbia River bar. When we were driving home, after leaving our friend and his boat at the marina, John asked, "Who was that man with us?"

I swallowed back my fear that his dementia was increasing at a faster pace than I anticipated and told myself that he would be okay. And for most of that summer, he was. Our son from Vancouver visited frequently and his other son and two of his daughters each came for a week. They were all able to go fishing with their father and were not alarmed by his forgetfulness, convinced, as I had once been, that his mental lapses were nothing more than normal aging.

In October 2015 John pulled his boat out of the water for the winter. By then, his driving was limited to trips to the marina or to the landfill, but he was still able to back the boat trailer into the water, maneuver his boat onto it, drive it home, and park boat and trailer in our boatshed. He could also handle his truck's manual transmission far better than me. He could no longer, however, back my friend's boat up her driveway, and his movements had become so slow that I began to question whether his reaction time while driving was fast enough to cope with an emergency situation, such as someone stopping suddenly in front of him. As if he sensed his own limitations, John now seemed content to let me drive wherever we needed to go, especially after November when we purchased a new car with an automatic transmission, and he couldn't figure out how to drive it.

Meanwhile my own health issues were beginning to affect my perspective on life. We were gradually withdrawing from social activities, partly because invitations were no longer forthcoming and partly because it was becoming too stressful for me to handle my own social anxiety and monitor John's growing confusion at the same time. It was becoming increasingly more difficult to cope with his incessant questions and his irritation when the answer wasn't immediately forthcoming, with the need for me to make every decision and take care of every crisis that arose in our daily lives and with the fear I felt every time I left him alone, not knowing if I would come back to a disaster. There were few hours in the day when I was not worried about something, and my emotions ranged from feeling sorry for myself and angry with John to condemning myself for being weak and intolerant and sometimes just plain lazy. In late 2015, after suffering from a bout of pneumonia and pleurisy brought on by stress and sheer exhaustion, I knew I could no longer carry this burden alone.

Reluctantly, I made an appointment with John's doctor who administered another MMSE test. The results were so low that he recommended another DriveAble test. Six years had passed since his last test, and this time, when John failed, I did not protest.

CAREGIVING

I live in a place of lost objects
Where plans are cast aside
And time is scattered like leaves upon the wind
Where there is no reasoning, no tolerance
From the one who needs it most.
Now, he says! It must be found now!
And I scream inside,
I don't care! I don't care!
All the while knowing that if I didn't care
I would not need to scream.

CHAPTER FIVE

Humour

RESISTANCE

"Put the scraps in the compost bucket," I tell you,
But you want to feed the dog we used to own.
Forgetting, no matter how often I tell you,
That the scraps will feed rats instead of dogs,
You sneak outside and happily scatter
Crumbs and crusts about the yard.
Subversive resistance, I call it.
You just think I'm nuts.

According to the Mayo Clinic, laughter provides both immediate and lasting health benefits. Besides increasing oxygen intake and the release of endorphins, it activates and relieves stress and soothes tension in our bodies. Over the longer term, laughter enhances our immune system, is a great pain reliever, makes it easier for us to cope with difficulties, and improves our moods.[1]

As a caregiver, I was constantly using humour to counteract the stress and frustration of living with a person with dementia, sometimes by making a conscious effort to find something to laugh about, but mostly because it was a lifelong habit. I grew up in a large family and times were often more than tough. Over the years we lost two homes and all our belongings to house fires. At the age of five, I was sent to a tuberculosis sanatorium and for eleven long months had no contact with anyone in my family except my mother. We moved often and more than once my mother scraped the bottom of the cupboard to feed us. We lost a lot, but the one thing we didn't lose and that saved us from being engulfed in despair was our ability to look at things from the funny side, even in some of our darkest moments.

My father was not an easy man to live with, but he adored my mother, and in the months following his death in 1999 she told me she often felt as if half of her was missing. A year later she, too, succumbed to cancer. Sitting outside that night, my siblings were reminiscing about her, trying to find in their memories a way to ease their hurting. One brother was watching a moth flitting about a deck lamp when a second moth arrived and instantly coupled with the first. "Well, Dad's found Mom," my brother quipped, and everyone roared with laughter. Anyone listening might be forgiven for thinking we were a callous lot, but all of us on that deck had put our lives and families and careers on hold to support Mom through her last painful weeks of battling cancer, and every one of us was feeling heartbroken and exhausted. But by allowing ourselves to see the humour of that moment, we were strengthened. Our laughter reminded us that there was still comedy in a world that had seemingly gone crazy, and although our mother was gone, joy in our memories of her was not.

There are many articles, such as "The Healing Power of Laughter in Death and Grief" by Marilyn A. Mendoza in *Psychology Today*[2], that emphasize the therapeutic benefits of humour when coping with grief and other challenges that life can throw at us. Deliberately choosing humour as a strategy is also the focus of "The Superpower of Humour," a TED talk by humourist and motivational speaker Judy Croon.[3] In their TED talk, "Why Great Leaders Take Humour Seriously," behavioural scientist Jennifer Aaker and corporate strategist Naomi Bagdonas[4] demonstrate how the use of humour can influence decision-makers and ease tense situations.

Even before I became a caregiver, focussing on the lighter side of a situation often saved me from murdering, destroying, or otherwise mutilating whoever or whatever happened to be within my reach, including my own self when things didn't go according to plan.

One day while courting me at Clowhom Falls, John had driven over the mountain to the shore where my float house was moored and offered to take me out to get firewood. Since my winter's supply was pretty meagre, I readily agreed and didn't realize until we were creeping along a logging road past a logged-off hillside where only slash remained, that he was also looking for a deer. It was hunting season and he had his rifle mounted above the rear truck window. As we started down a long switchback, he suddenly spied a huge buck on the other side of the ravine, and in mere seconds he'd parked, grabbed his rifle, and taken aim. The rifle cracked and the buck went down.

"Bring the truck around," he called over his shoulder then headed down into the ravine and up the other side.

I had never driven his truck and was terrified of the steep, unstable backroads, but I clearly had no choice. Holding my breath, I drove down and around the corner and up the other side of the ravine, stopping the truck at a spot I thought was just above where the buck had been standing and then made my way down through the slash to help him. The deer was so huge he had to cut it in two in order for us to carry it to the truck, and we were both sweating hard by the time it was safely stored in the bed. John, obviously very proud of his prowess, was beaming at the huge rack of antlers when I said quietly, "I don't think it's going to burn very well."

Startled, he turned to me. "Burn?"

"Well, we *were* getting firewood, weren't we?"

He laughed, and I think it was then he decided I was the woman he wanted to marry.

John, too, had used humour to avoid conflict. Once after enduring a hot day on the golf course with my father, who insisted that he would love this sport, John quietly turned in his clubs.

"So, how did you like it?" Dad asked, expecting an enthusiastic response.

With a deadpan expression, my fisherman husband said, "It was okay . . . but how do you cook 'em?"

Dad looked at him questioningly.

"The golfs," John explained with deliberate patience. "I can't figure out how you're going to cook them."

My father wasn't impressed, but John howled, and he delighted in retelling the story whenever the subject of golf came up.

Sometimes the humour of a caregiving disaster surfaced when I was writing in my journal. After one particularly trying day, when I was dealing with a rat that had invaded our home, my supply of patience ran dry, and I lashed out at John who was doing nothing except being John. *John asked if he could help*, I wrote that night, *and I bit his head off. It lies in shreds on the kitchen floor.* It didn't save John, but it did ease my distress about being so mean.

Often my own foibles provided the humour I needed to get through a rough patch. One day when I was already feeling cranky and out of sorts, I stopped at the cardlock where I gas-up my car and discovered a new challenge. The cardlock had only one set of pumps and both the north and south access lanes to them were empty, so it should have been easy for me to drive up and fill my tank. But when I got out, I discovered my tank was on the opposite side of the car to the pump. Frustrated, I drove around the pumps and once again stepped out to fuel the tank—only the tank was still on the opposite side to the pumps. Seriously wondering if it was I, and not John, who was suffering from dementia, I stood studying the pumps and my car, trying to determine how I had to maneuver the car to position my fuel tank next to the pumps. I'd like to say here that I figured it out, but it wasn't until I ended up on the wrong side one more time that I gave up driving around the pumps and, instead, drove back to the street and started from my usual entrance that I finally lined up tank to pump and was able to obtain the fuel. Hoping no one had noticed my moment of insanity, I left the cardlock and headed home, and it was as I was driving that the hilarity of my run-in with the pumps struck me. I started to laugh and did not stop until I drove into the yard. By then I'd lost every molecule of crankiness and was able to enjoy the rest of my day.

When they aren't driving us crazy, I've found children are an endless source of amusement, and occasionally the humour I needed came from my granddaughter. One summer afternoon when she and her cousin were visiting, I found my stress levels were rising as I tried to cope with them and John's impatience with their noise and the confusion it was causing him. The girls were fascinated by the smaller wildlife inhabiting our yard and were happily engaged in catching and examining an assortment of bugs, beetles, and snails, when Granddaughter suddenly exclaimed, "OMG! I've got a pregnant red ant!"

Her cousin immediately picked it up, then grew frightened, and dropped it in her shoe. The two started shrieking until the ant was retrieved and placed in their bug box. Studying the discarded shoe, Granddaughter observed, "I think it pooped in your shoe."

I wisely refrained from asking how my granddaughter determined that the ant was pregnant. As I chuckled over their conversation, my stress levels dropped.

Humour is a useful tool even for persons with dementia. One day we were visiting in a park with friends, one of whom didn't disguise his irritation at John's slow way of telling a very long story. John grew quiet after that, but when he had to go to the washroom, he stood and instead of using the walking poles that helped him with his balance, he handed them to me and, holding his arms out like a tightrope walker, comically staggered towards the washrooms. Even our irritated friend couldn't help but laugh.

John also used humour to hide the fact that he couldn't remember something. One night as we sat watching television, he said wistfully, "I sure wish I knew what happened to our dog."

Since we had owned several dogs in the past, and it had been more than a year since we'd given away our last pet, I asked, "Which one?"

He looked at me straight-faced and said, "The one we don't see anymore."

During an assessment, his case worker asked John what his address was. He said, "Here." When she asked him what day it was, he said, "The day after the one that just passed."

One day he came down to breakfast all out of sorts.

"What's wrong?" I asked.

"They keep saying I have to leave," he said morosely.

For once, instead of being angry that he should have such troubling thoughts, I saw the humour in the situation and responded with mock sternness, "Well, you tell 'they' that I'm your wife and I say you're not going anywhere!"

He smiled gratefully, his good humour restored.

In "Finding the Funny in Crummy,"[5] a TEDxBeaconStreet Talk, humourist Amy Lyle addresses not just the healing power of humour but also how humour helps us to connect with each other, something very useful to know when trying to interact with a partner suffering from dementia. One evening as we sat on the couch, John looked deep into my eyes and asked me to marry him. He was astonished and delighted when I said we were already married and showed him our wedding photos. "I've never been happier in my life!" he exclaimed, and I felt a small satisfaction.

After all the years of coming in second, I had finally beat out the fish in his life.

Sometimes it takes a super-conscious effort for us to find something to laugh or even smile about, especially when we are up to our necks in the caregiver swamp and fighting off one alligator after another. But humour truly is all around us. It can be found on a television sitcom or a humour site on the Internet. Type "jokes" into the search engine and you can be engaged for hours reading or watching jokes. Free video lessons on the benefits of laughter yoga can be found by Googling "laughter yoga" or by visiting www.laughteryogacanada.org.

When all else fails, we can look back on our day and deliberately search for the moments that caused us to smile—even if the only thing we find is a pregnant ant.

SEAGULL BUTT

I'm looking at a seagull's butt.
Translucent tail feathers fan
In silent applause
For causing poop to cascade
Upon my head.
Is the lesson in this
That all beauty is followed
By crap?
Or that above the crap
Beauty reigns?

CHAPTER SIX

Getting Help

IF I COULD DO IT AGAIN

If I could do it all again, I would seek help sooner,
Create a caring circle of family, friends, and paid help,
Discover everything I could about the progression
And demands of this disease, and become best buddies
With community organizations and the health care system.

If I had to do it all again, I would augment my stock
Of humour and resilience with inspirational music,
Philosophies and reference books, and attend
A multitude of workshops, seminars, and support groups,
Arming myself with knowledge, strategies, and self-esteem.

If I had to do it all again, I would let go of my
Overinflated ego that insists that I'm the only one
Who can do this job right, and appreciate that others
Can, in their own way, make a positive difference
To the well-being of the one who is in need of care.

I would do this not because I'm lazy or lack devotion,
Or feel sorry for myself, or am an inadequate human.
I would do this because it is the only way to reduce harm
And enhance my ability to be kind and supportive,
And the best that I can be for the one that I love most.

As soon as they heard of John's dementia, my friends and family reached out.

"Let us know what we can do," they said. "We are here for you."

I knew they spoke from the heart, that their offers were sincere, and even today I am not sure why I resisted this help or why other caregivers do the same. For me, it probably had something to do with my exaggerated sense of responsibility for others and my lack of self esteem. I'd always felt obliged to be the one who provided care and support, and if I failed to do so, I didn't have the right to walk on this planet, to breathe its air, or accept its gifts. Other caregivers have told me they just felt it was what they had to do to honour marriage vows or to look after a parent or sibling or sometimes a friend.

"I wasn't opposed to the idea of getting help," one caregiver told me, "but when my partner objected to strangers in the house, I didn't want to upset her. I could manage."

It wasn't until I became ill and had no other choice that I finally accepted help from others. I realized that if I was hospitalized or died, the man I loved would be left with no one to stand with him as his dementia progressed. But instead of complete surrender, I set up an elaborate, internal accounting system wherein I'd accept someone's help then spend hours figuring out how I could pay them back with gifts or future favours. I could share my skills and labour, I told myself, even though every skill and every moment I had was already in the red by several years. I was using resources I would desperately need later, eating the seeds in the winter that I would need for planting in the spring, so to speak. For someone already suffering from chronic anxiety, this looming bankruptcy of resources, whether real or imagined, was like living on the edge of a cliff that could crumble at any moment. Night after night I lay sleeplessly tossing and turning and staring at the ceiling, waiting for the cliff to disintegrate.

As much as I needed help, I also needed a greater understanding of dementia, so I attended another workshop sponsored by the Alzheimer Society of BC. Although this one was about a more advanced dementia than John was currently exhibiting, I did learn about windows—moments of clarity that can last for minutes, hours, or even days. Seemingly out of the blue, even people with advanced dementia can remember names, where they are, what day it is, and how to do things that they've been finding impossible. In contrast, John's "windows" seemed more like dementia windows. He functioned normally most of the time and his occasional slips into dementia, such as the one on our friend's boat, would only last for an hour or, at the most, a day.

I also learned about sundowning, a term used to describe the confusion, agitation, and aggression that many persons with dementia experience later in the day. This can be present in the early stages of dementia but is more prevalent during the middle stages.

According to the instructor, one of the hardest lessons to learn when dealing with this disease is that there is no point in arguing with someone suffering from dementia. Their brains simply can't let go of an idea once they've fixated on it, and trying to make them do so only frustrates everyone involved. The best solution, she said, is to create a distraction—suggest a treat, an activity, or anything that will shift their attention. This isn't easy, in part because the same distraction often doesn't work more than once or twice. Coming up with something that does work takes time and patience, but it also reduces the angry explosions that result from a caregiver who insists that something must be done "right" or that an inaccurate statement has to be corrected. What the person with dementia is saying could be a thousand miles from accurate, but to them it is real and makes perfect sense and they are no longer able to understand that it isn't.

Dementia, I discovered, is a scary place to be. Those suffering from it don't know that they can't remember; they only know that the people closest to them are suddenly acting very strangely, and although they sense that something is wrong, they can't figure out what it is. They do, however, sense the reactions of the people around them, and while they may forget the angry or sarcastic words directed at them, they do not forget how that person made them feel. I noticed that visitors whose remarks or behaviour were hurtful to John, even if their intention was not to harm, were suddenly on the list of people he didn't want to be around. He couldn't remember why. He just became angry or afraid when they were around.

I went home from the workshop resolved to be stronger, more resilient, and most of all, more patient with my husband. Saint Rosella, at your service! Needless to say, I failed miserably. Wallowing in guilt and shame after having a hissy fit over John's insistence that we had to empty the ashes before lighting the heater, even though we'd emptied them just a few days earlier, I meekly accepted a referral from John's doctor to the Alzheimer Society's First Link program, and to the Older Adult Mental Health (OAMH) service.

On a cold and rainy day in November 2015, Kathy Thomas, an OAMH psychiatric nurse, ushered me into her tiny office. Not sure what to expect, I took a seat and waited while she settled into her own chair. She was a kindly lady about my own age, and she spoke so gently and caringly that I found myself sobbing out my story. Undeterred by my tears, she handed me a box of Kleenex and assured me this was a common reaction from caregivers who were emotionally and physically drained.

"I feel so hopeless," I said. "It's as if doors are closing on me left and right. And I'm resentful. John has lived a full life doing what he wanted. I have lived mine doing what other people wanted. Looking after my siblings, my parents, my child. Now John. By the time this is over, I will be too old to do any of the things I thought I'd do after I retired."

Kathy held my hand as I told her how lonely I was, how I was no longer able to talk to John about the problems with the house or my fears and frustrations. He would not understand most of it, and what he might understand would only make him feel terrible.

"He was my best friend and my partner, and we did everything together. Now, doing the simplest thing with him is so frustrating I want to scream!" Just the thought of this caused me to shift from tears to anger. "He moves so slowly, and I must adapt to his pace because he can't speed up. If we're walking and I start thinking about something else, I am soon charging ahead of him. When I notice this, I have to stop and wait and try not to let him see my annoyance. Sometimes I think I'm going to explode, and then I am ashamed because he is working so hard just to move, and his knee is hurting and yet he doesn't give up.

"I feel so scared," I said, "that I won't be able to give John what he needs, or I will say or do something that hurts him, or that I will hate him. And I can't bear to think of him not being here. Even with his dementia, he is still my rock. I love him. I want to be with him. And I want to be me. I hate what is happening. I hate whining and feeling sorry for myself. Most of all, I hate being so bloody, bloody tired!"

When I had poured out my heart, Kathy gently assured me that everything I was feeling was normal, that I was responding in a very human way to the enormous challenges I was facing. She had been there herself, she said, had dealt with her husband's dementia until his death. It was a hard journey even for someone who'd spent her career looking after mentally compromised patients, but there was help available.

"Why don't you come to our caregiver support group?" she suggested. "We meet once a week right here. It's very informal and

I think you will receive a lot of comfort and support from being with other caregivers."

I left her office with a tiny seed of hope planted in my chest. Nothing had changed in my situation, but my perspective had shifted ever so slightly.

The following Wednesday I attended my first caregiver support group meeting. There were almost a dozen caregivers there, mostly women. One by one they introduced themselves and told their stories—some were caring for a parent, others for a spouse. They had been meeting together for several years, and I sensed a caring and openness among them as they shared, sometimes in tears, the difficulties they'd encountered over the past week or funny incidents that made us laugh. One person told of how her spouse in late-stage dementia had tried to toast a cell phone.

At first I felt like an outsider, but they welcomed me warmly and encouraged me to share as little or as much of my story as I wanted. I did not break down as I had in the nurse's office, and I was able to give an overview of my situation and some of the issues I was facing. Many of them gave a "been there, done that" nod that was oddly reassuring.

"We're a wacky group," someone said, "but we care. Coming here, being able to talk with others who know exactly what we're going through has saved our lives."

As I walked back to my car, I felt better. That seed of hope was sprouting, though it was still far below the surface.

A week later I contacted the First Link Dementia Helpline, as John's doctor had advised, and John and I were invited to attend a Minds in Motion (MIM) class, "a fitness and social program designed for persons with early-stage dementia along with a family member, friend or other care partner."[6]

"It's for people with early-stage dementia and their caregivers," I told John.

This meant nothing to him since he didn't believe he had dementia, but he agreed to go with me.

"I love you," he said, "and I love being with you. So long as you're there, I'm happy."

Not knowing what to expect, I led the way to a small room at the Sechelt recreation centre. Gathered there were several couples. Like the caregivers in the support group, they had the easy, relaxed way of people who have known each other for a long time. Lori, the co-ordinator of the program, welcomed us warmly, introduced us to the others and then hustled everyone to the gym for the exercise part of the program.

Once we were all seated on chairs in a circle that took up most of the gym, Lori explained that the low impact exercises were designed to help seniors maintain their mobility, especially their ability to get on and off a toilet without assistance. "One of the reasons that seniors end up in a care home," she said, "is because they are no longer able to use the toilet." To my chagrin, while John seemed to catch on quite quickly to the exercises, I required several instances of one-on-one instruction, partly because I've never been able to distinguish between left and right.

The exercises were followed by a game with a ball. There was much laughter and a camaraderie among both caregivers and "participants" as those with dementia were called. When this session was complete, we all met again in the small room for coffee or tea and a cookie, and then sat at tables of four or five for a game of bingo. The games were different every week, sometimes involving cards or dice or listing various things, such as objects in a kitchen or a garden. The point was not to win, but to have fun, to interact, and to provide mental stimulation for the person with dementia.

As we walked away from the rec centre, I asked John if he'd enjoyed himself, and he nodded with enthusiasm. "They seem like very nice people," he said and readily agreed to attend the next class.

On a different day, Lori also taught a "Move Strong Keep Fit" exercise class that she suggested might benefit John and leave me free for an hour to do whatever I wanted. Surprisingly, John agreed to this, too, without any persuasion, and as it turned out, that hour was just enough time for me to have a good workout on the treadmill in the weight room adjoining the gym.

Just as I was getting used to the support group and MIM classes, we were into the Christmas season, a time that has always been stressful for me. My expectations of myself to create a perfect holiday had always exceeded the limitations of my time, energy, and abundance. This year the stress was even worse as I tried to look after John, entertain my granddaughter and her cousin with craft projects and decorating gingerbread cookies and houses, attend Christmas parties with John or alone (which meant arranging for someone to stay with him), bake endless cookies and bars to use as Christmas gifts, and prepare for a visit from John's daughter, her husband and son. "No" just didn't seem to be among the words in my vocabulary, and as the season wore on, my anxiety levels reached record peaks.

Among the parties I attended was one with the caregiver support group. Still not sure of my commitment to the group, I prepared a plate of cookies and bars and ventured forth. There were more people than usual in attendance, most of whom I did not know, but as before, they were all friendly and welcoming. Everything seemed to be going well with stories shared and much laughter—until it came time for a group photo. The sun was shining through a window that was behind both the group and a table that was laden with the stereo providing Christmas music, a basket of gifts to be distributed to everyone, a couple of plates with lingering lunch remains and a few glasses of punch. While others discussed ways and means to access and close the window blinds, I, ever the helpful one, said, "No problem!" Clearing a corner of the table, I climbed onto it and reached for the blinds. Only the table legs had not been properly secured and as I stretched forward, the whole thing collapsed beneath me. While others rescued the gifts from the spilled drinks, I, red-faced and mortified, stumbled to a chair, and remained there, as I should have done in the first place, until the picture was taken. A few minutes later I escaped to my car, vowing never to return.

Of course, I did return. I had no choice.

I am afraid, I wrote in my journal. *Afraid of losing control. Afraid of me. Afraid of the future. I say I don't care. I don't want to live. And the next moment I'm dialing the medical clinic! I want to stop wanting. I want to feel good again, to feel like running, to be hopeful about tomorrow, to hear music, or read a passage in a book and feel uplifted or enlightened. I see myself isolated and alienated from everyone because I have nothing to offer any more.*

One morning, I asked John if he was happy. He said sometimes. He also said I was his bright spot, that I took care of him and helped him manage things.

"I love you," he said. "I love being with you."

We hugged and laughed a little, and someone looking on would say all was right with our world.

The constant tug-of-war between laughing and crying was so confusing, and it occurred to me that it is not just the person with dementia who changes from day to day. I was changing as well, and I didn't like the changes in me any more than I liked the changes in John.

Desperate for anything that might shift these thoughts, I forced myself to attend the next support group, and this time broke down in front of everyone, just as I had done in Kathy's office. The group was sympathetic and understanding because each person there had been in the exact position at some point in their caregiving journey. When the session was over, the coordinator, Jane, took me aside.

"We have a new psychiatrist on staff," she said, "and his patient list is still small. He might be able to help you. If you like, I'll speak with him."

I gave a feeble nod. Anything, I thought, was better than the pain and exhaustion and overwhelming hopelessness that had become my life.

The Alzheimer Society also sponsored a caregiver support group that met in the evening on the first Wednesday of every month. Many of those attending were also enrolled in the Minds in Motion program. Since John was usually content to watch television at that time of night, and I felt safe leaving him alone for two hours, I signed on. The majority of caregivers attending this group were men, and I found this helpful because it gave me a male perspective on John's situation, enabling me to better understand how my actions might be affecting him.

Opening up about myself at support groups seemed to have opened a tap that wouldn't shut off, and on my first visit to the psychiatrist that Jane had arranged for me to see, I divulged much more of my life than I intended. I was momentarily relieved by his assurance that, while he could not change what I was feeling, he could offer insights that would help me cope better with those feelings, but that evening my relief shifted to anxiety and fear.

I feel exposed and very afraid, I wrote in my journal. *I want to curl up in a ball under my desk or bed or in a dark closet. To hide away.* All night long, bits of our conversation—mostly my words—kept running through my mind. *How could I have said that? What must he think of me?* Needless to say, I slept little.

By the following day, however, feeling stronger and more determined, I took stock of my situation. John had dementia. Besides caring for him, I had seemingly endless social and family obligations, a book to write, a business to manage and an emotional history that needed to be acknowledged and dealt with. At the same time, I had strength and with the support groups and doctors to lean on, I also had the beginnings of hope.

THE SUPPORT GROUP

We begin as strangers,
Afraid at first,
Wary of revealing our sins,
Scared to express our pain
And confusion,
Believing we will unleash
A flood of misery
That cannot be contained.

Slowly . . . as we hear the stories
And feel the anguish
Of others
We are drawn in . . . begin to trust and to share
And the burden grows less heavy;
We even smile
And sometimes laugh
And go home feeling
As if we can bear tomorrow.

Then we begin to care,
To worry if someone doesn't show,
To weep when someone shares a hurting
Worse than our own,
To feel the loss
When a loved one declines
Or dies;
Yet in our sadness for them
Is the fear . . . *Will I be the next to stand in their shoes?*

We become a family,
Brothers and sisters bound by fate
And a cruel disease that leaves
No one standing;
In our togetherness
Is strength;
In our shared loss a comfort
And in our hearts the knowing
That we are not alone.

CHAPTER SEVEN

Inspiration

LIFT ME UP

Lift me up from the river,
Lift me up from the sea,
Lift me up from my sorrows,
Lead me from this misery.

Lift me up in the gloaming,
Lift me up in the night,
Lift me up in the morning,
Let me walk into the light.

Lift me up from the heartache,
Lift me up from my pain,
Lift me up from my struggle,
Lift me up to start again.

Lift me up so I can dance,
Lift me up so I can fly,
Lift me up so that my song,
Will reach beyond the sky.

Lift me up from the river,
Lift me up from the sea,
Lift me up from my sorrows,
Let me be all I can be

I've discovered that sources of comfort, positive messages, and inspiration exist all around me, but sometimes, though they are dispatched with love and the best of intentions, they arrive on a day when positivity is the last thing I want to read or hear. On these occasions I have been sorely tempted to send the bearer of the cheery, look-on-the-bright-side message flying butt-first into the darkest side of hell. Of course, once my anger dissipates, such thoughts shift to shame, and guilt being a great motivator, I do penance by digging deeper into the message, often finding something that does lift my spirits. My doctors, therapist, support groups, agencies such as the Alzheimer Society or Older Adult Mental Health, TED Talks and other online videos, have also provided me with insights that helped me to survive the worst of times.

Much of my anxiety, I learned, was caused by erroneous sub-conscious beliefs, and slowly I came to understand it was possible to counteract these beliefs with conscious truths. New thoughts create new neural pathways in the amygdala portion of the brain—the part that initiates the fight-or-flight reaction—and over time as these pathways grow stronger, our automatic reaction to circumstances can be shifted from panic (fight-or-flight) to a simple acknowledgement that something is amiss. Without the panic, the rational part of the brain is then free to deal with the issue at hand. My psychiatrist (aka therapist) explained that, though my original subconscious beliefs will always be there, I can counteract them with new thoughts.

One of the distorted beliefs I deal with is that bad things happen because I'm not good enough or clever enough or generous enough—or just plain not enough. As ridiculous as it sounds, when John developed dementia, I felt I was to blame. Eventually I challenged this belief by acknowledging that dementia results from physical changes in a person's brain, and by asking myself how exactly could I have caused this to happen? Did I reach inside John's head and physically manipulate his brain? Did I feed or inject him with a substance that would physically change his brain? The answer was consistently no. Later, I was introduced to a mantra that showed I was not alone in taking responsibility for a disease far beyond my control—the three "Cs" that every dementia caregiver needs to learn: *I did not cause it, I cannot cure it, and I cannot control it.* By repeating this message again and again, I gradually trained my subconscious brain to stop panicking every time I made a mistake or got angry or said something to John that I wished I hadn't. Instead, I began to understand that while my action might have resulted in a moment or two of discomfort or sadness for him, it had done nothing to cause or intensify his dementia.

We cannot stop catastrophic things from happening to ourselves or to those dear to us, but many of us employ drastic measures such as fear or guilt to try to accomplish this impossibility. I could use my fear of being called a coward, for example, to motivate myself to walk across a high bridge, the guilt I feel for being cross with John today to stop myself from being cross with him tomorrow. But there are healthier ways to motivate my behaviour, such as reassuring myself that I have the physical and mental fitness required to walk safely across the bridge, and that the bridge's stability is tested on a regular basis. By reminding myself of times when I have been patient with John, I can stop condemning myself for being cross today and focus on doing better tomorrow. The difference in the two ways of approaching the same difficulty are subtle, but the shift in how I feel afterwards is huge.

One of the hardest emotional reactions I had to deal with as a caregiver was the feeling that I was in a prison from which there was no exit. In *Man's Search for Meaning*, Viktor Frankl, a neurologist, psychiatrist, and philosopher who survived the Holocaust, quotes Friedrich Nietzsche: "He who has a why to live for can bear almost any how." For me finding that "why," however, was not easy, especially when my mind was fogged with grief, anger, depression, and exhaustion. On days when the fog lifted slightly, I would say that my "why" was writing and being present for my son and granddaughter if they needed me and, of course, for looking after John. When I concentrated on those things, I was encouraged to keep going.

The "why" is unique to each of us, and sometimes the light it shines is almost too dim to see, but it is there. Frankl credits his survival in the camps to finding his "why"—to use his experiences and observations to help others and to develop his theory of logotherapy (a form of psychotherapy "based on the premise that the primary motivational force of an individual is to find meaning in life.")[7] He believed that meaning and hidden opportunities can be found in any challenge, suffering or misfortune. "In the concentration camps, for example, in this living laboratory and on this testing ground, we watched and witnessed some of our comrades behaving like swine while others behaved like saints. Man has both potentialities within himself; which one is actualized depends on decisions but not on conditions."[8] A great part of my caregiving experience was coping with depression, a condition, according to Frankl's theory, that occurs when people are faced with tasks beyond their abilities, diminished energy, and the realization that they are not the persons they believe they should be. On good days I was able to appreciate that, while I would never have dreamed that I had the inner resources to look after someone who often could not even remember my name, never mind how to turn on the shower, I was, in fact, doing just that. Bad, good, or otherwise, it did not matter—I was caring for my husband. On even better days, I found ways to ensure that I was rested—arranging for family or friends and sometimes paid help to take over the job long enough for me to replenish my energy reserves. When the voice in my head nagged me about being the worst caregiver in the world, I countered with a single, true statement: I'm doing the best that I possibly can, and absolutely no one can ask for more than that. And even more significantly: I am here. I am doing it. That is enough.

Another Holocaust survivor, Dr. Edith Eger, author of two books, *The Gift* and *The Choice*, helped me when it seemed like there would be no end to the sadness and frustration and hopelessness that dominated the half-life I was living as a caregiver. Her message that "I go through the valley of the shadow of death. I don't camp there"[9] helped reinforce the truth that nothing in life lasts forever and, as my therapist often reminded me, "This, too, shall pass." By not cementing my attention only on the hard parts of losing John and caring for someone with dementia, I could also appreciate the good parts—those rare moments when we were still able to be close and intimate, despite the dementia, the beautiful way he smiled and the eagerness with which he greeted an opportunity to go for a walk or a drive. I also discovered resilience in myself that I never knew was there. Although my physical health declined because of the stress, my determination and ingenuity grew stronger with every challenge I met and conquered. "Our painful experiences aren't a liability, they are a gift," writes Dr. Eger. "They give us perspective and meaning, an opportunity to find our unique purpose and our strength."[10] TED Talks, other online videos, and books also helped to lift my spirits. I would type into the search engine words such as "videos on happiness" or "how to cope with frustration?" or "ways to deal with anger" or simply, "grieving." Each search resulted in a generous selection of videos that explored the issue and offered fresh ways of coping. Many echoed or provided a different version of the ideas put forth in the works of Viktor Frankl and Edith Eger.

A TED Talk given by physicist Neil Hughes not only helped me deal with some of the anxiety I was experiencing but also made me laugh. His three-part strategy called "A new plan for anxious feelings: escape the custard!" begins with noticing our thought patterns, especially negative thoughts that he compares to invisible "pudding traps." He advises that when such unwanted thoughts happen, he tries to do something different, such as, "Stand up and sing the Danish national anthem. It won't help. Not least because I don't know the Danish national anthem, but it will break me out of the loop I'm in."[11] His third strategy is to replace habitual thoughts with a positive thought. In my own case, that could mean shifting the thought that *I'm a terrible caregiver (or wife or daughter or whatever)* to *I love my husband/mother/friend with all my heart, and I am doing the best I know how to help.*

One of the top twenty TEDx Talks in 2020 was Lucy Hone's "The Three Secrets of Resilient People." Hone had worked through her own grief over the loss of her twelve-year-old daughter, and her advice really hit home for me as I dealt with the gradual loss of my husband. Her three secrets begin with recognizing that suffering is a part of life and is not directed at any particular person. I was not being punished, nor did I "deserve" John's dementia any more than he was being punished or deserved dementia. It happened. (Hone found herself not asking "Why me?" but "Why not me?"). Her second secret is to tune out the negative news that we are bombarded with every day by media and other sources and direct our attention to what is still good around us. She describes how, on a day when she was overwhelmed by doubts, she thought, "You cannot get swallowed up by this—you've got so much to live for. Don't lose what you have to what you have lost." The third secret of resilient people, she maintains, is to notice what you are doing and ask yourself, "Is what I am doing [or thinking] helping or harming me?" By asking this simple question, she says, "you're putting yourself back in the driver's seat. It gives you control over your decision-making."[12] When I asked myself that question,

I often came to realize that what I was doing was definitely not helping me, and I was able to do something different.

Some of the videos I watched and books I read worked for me; others didn't. The usefulness of the message could last a few minutes or hours or days. Sometimes I would forget and have to read or view the message again. Each one provided me with something that strengthened my resolve and enabled me to get through another day, to accept something I could not change, devise a plan of action that I could focus on, and gave me a tiny fragment of hope that there might be a smile waiting when this caregiving journey was over.

Learning more about caring for someone with dementia also helped to inspire me and gave me something concrete to do. There are many online resources, such as the Alzheimer Society of Canada, with easy-to-understand information about the disease of dementia, helpful strategies for caring for someone with dementia, and (most important for me when the caregiving got harder than I could manage on my own) an entire section devoted to reducing caregiver stress.[13] Teepa Snow's videos on caring for someone with dementia were helpful not only for understanding the disease but also for their practical advice on caregiving and dealing with the feelings of both the person with dementia and the caregiver.[14]

Sometimes all it took to shift the mood for me was a visit to Starbucks. Escaping there for an hour of alone time, I would treat myself to a chai latte and settle in for some serious writing. For some reason, the chatter from other customers and the music slipped into the background and for that brief time I was fulfilled. Sometimes I even wrote whimsical poems, such as "The Sign."

This doesn't mean that there were not times when I felt overwhelmed, when I was reacting emotionally to circumstance rather than choosing my reaction. When this happened, I clung to the belief that this storm would also pass, and when it did, I would get up, dry or dust myself off, and begin again with renewed spirit.

THE SIGN

The sign blink-blinking in the window
Cries out, "See me! See me!"
Begging, beckoning, beseeching
Passersby to enter,
To purchase,
To enable the sign
To keep blink-blinking in the window.

CHAPTER EIGHT

Guilt Selfcare And Boundaries

DAILY CHORE

He walks slowly,
Minus two kilometres per hour,
Placing one foot doggedly
In front of the other,
Ignoring the pain,
And my chatter.
Occasionally he stops,
Looks out at the clouds
Or the water birds.
"Is that a ship?" he asks.
"It's Seagull Island," I say.
"You used to fish there."
He walks to the edge
Of the embankment
Where there is no railing
To stop a fall,
And peers down,
Confident that his poles
Will hold him steady.
They are a double-edged sword,
These Nordic sticks of shame,
That he both hates and needs.
He walks the distance

Then click-clicks back to the car
Tired but proud.
Blind to the courage of his steps,
I grumble about this daily chore.
It is not my finest hour.

Guilt is a harsh taskmaster. As John's dementia progressed and my emotional stability wavered, that taskmaster came to govern more and more of my life. "No" seemed to have been lost from my vocabulary, and I was sacrificing myself to both this guilt and my (erroneous) belief that it was my responsibility to look after everyone else but me.

In early January 2016, six years after his diagnosis, John and I spent two days in Vancouver. We stayed one night with our son and his family in an apartment not designed for five people, especially not one suffering from dementia and unable to cope with the distraction of television, people he didn't recognize, and an energetic granddaughter. The second night we stayed with my sister and her husband. Her home was much quieter, but there was a steep stairwell down to our bedroom, and I was in constant fear of John falling as he made his way up or down. Disoriented by the changes to his routine, he was more confused than usual, and by the time we reached the ferry terminal to return home my stress levels were steadily rising.

"Oh, crap! The ferry is already in!" I cried as we stepped from the bus and hurried to the ticket booths. We were able to purchase our tickets, so I knew we would get on the ferry, but I also knew that if the upper ramp closed before we got to the gate, we would have to go down a steep stairway and board via the lower car deck. As we began to meet the passengers who had disembarked from the incoming ferry, I grew even more anxious. John was moving as fast as he could, but he was still agonizingly slow, and as I watched him struggle, I had to bite my tongue to keep from urging him to walk faster. It was my fault that we were late, not his, I told myself. I was in charge, and I had failed. Ashamed, I gritted my teeth and patted his shoulder.

"It's okay," I said encouragingly, concentrating on my steps instead of the long passage ahead. "We're doing just fine." Still, I almost cried from relief when we finally reached the departure gate and found the ramp still in place.

It took a few days after that trip for John to get back to what was his current "normal." It took me much longer to let go of my guilt for putting him in so many disorienting situations. That guilt, however, didn't stop me from continuing to volunteer my time and energies to causes I felt were more important than my own.

One of these causes was publicizing information about caregiver services that were available in the community, including how to access these services. Had my doctor not taken time from his busy schedule to learn about the OAMH clinic and steered me (and others) to Kathy Thomas, I might never have received the help I had so desperately needed. Many in our support group, including myself, had no idea how to connect with a caseworker, and we hadn't known that, without a caseworker, we could not access more advanced services. There was also a gap between what was being offered and what caregivers needed.

To address these gaps, our evening caregiver group decided to arrange a workshop, inviting both caregivers and service providers to come together to discuss what was needed and how those needs could be met. Brian Smith and I were co-facilitators, and we were soon busy gathering materials, preparing notices, and helping to set up the room we'd obtained for the event. We were pleased with the turnout and the enthusiasm of the caregivers attending, and when it was over, we crafted a letter outlining local caregiver needs and sent it to multiple agencies that we thought might help to address those needs. Those who attended the work-shop were so pleased to have had their concerns recognized that they wanted more, and a few months later we were arranging a second workshop.

At the same time I was also working on my latest novel; managing two rental units; looking after our extensive flower, berry, and vegetable gardens; caring for and entertaining my granddaughter when she visited; helping a friend to launch her boat then set out with her to check our crab traps; and looking after John's increasing needs. At night, instead of congratulating myself for my accomplishments, I lamented everything I hadn't accomplished, and my journal entries were boringly consistent: *Today was not productive. I should have done more.*

One summer day, although I was feeling miserable, I honoured a promise to go fishing with John. Pushing my pain aside, I managed to fake enough enthusiasm that he was happy with the trip, but by the time we reached home, I had developed a fever and my lower abdominal pain was so severe that I left him cleaning the fish we had caught and drove to Emergency. I was diagnosed with diverticulitis and given intravenous antibiotics before being discharged at two in the morning. A sane person would have taken this as a sign that rest was needed. Instead, I rose early to clean the house and make a special lunch for friends from California who were stopping by for a visit. By the time our friends left, I was worn out and spent the rest of the day lying on the couch. *I feel guilty for not cleaning up the dishes or watering the garden*, I wrote that night, *and all afternoon the word "lazy" came frequently to mind.*

As John's dementia progressed, he wanted to be with me every minute of the day—a condition of dementia referred to as "shadowing." He would be in the kitchen when I was making a meal or sitting in my office when I was writing or standing behind me when

I was working in the yard. Realizing that he was acting this way because he was feeling lost and vulnerable, I would attempt to distract him by giving him a task, but he usually couldn't understand the task, forgetting instructions as fast as I gave them, and I would need to repeat them and repeat them until I felt like screaming. In bed at night, when I usually loved to curl up beside him, savouring his warmth and our togetherness, I was now finding myself unable to breathe. The only way I could get any rest at all was to wait until he was asleep then make my escape to the bed in the guest room.

Sleeping with John, I wrote in my journal, *is an extension of the day. A part of me is still aware of him and his needs. When I sleep alone, I re-energize. It is a break from caregiving.*

I misinterpreted this as a betrayal of our marriage vows, and to counteract the guilt I was feeling, I would rise early and return to our bed before John woke. Or, if I heard him moving about in the night, I would go back to our bed to reassure him that all was well.

Sex was a constant source of guilt. As John's dementia progressed, his sexual appetite increased, while mine disappeared, and an act that was once a joyous release that resulted in a comforting closeness became a physically painful obligation. When, out of duty, I looked after his needs, I felt as if I had betrayed myself. When I refused him, I was overcome with guilt. Occasionally, if I felt I had neglected him or if I had lost my temper with him, sex was my act of penitence. He was happy regardless of my reason.

Sometimes I was able to override my sense of duty. When I needed to travel to the Cariboo to conduct research for the novel I was writing, I hired our friend, Patti, to stay with John. She is an energetic, cheerful person who thought of John almost as a second father. They shared a love for fishing and gathering wood and evenings by the fire talking about the past. Even so, he wasn't happy about being left behind.

John cried this morning about my going away, I wrote in my journal, *but after I showed him where I was going and gave him a copy of the course I'm taking, he said he felt better. I felt guilty about leaving him, but I am determined to do this. I am so tired, and though I don't know if this will help, it surely cannot hurt. As I drove away from home, down the deserted road, I felt like a bird being released from a cage.*

For the most part, however, guilt was my constant companion. I was doing too much for others and neglecting John. I wasn't doing enough for anyone. I was ignoring friends, or I was spending too much time with friends. I was forcing John to endure some event just so I could attend, or I was leaving him out by not taking him with me. After cancelling a planned fishing trip with him because of an erroneous wind warning, I wrote: *Feeling guilty about not going fishing. The water was calm, but I was tired, and my frozen shoulder was hurting. I have disappointed everyone.* When I did push my tiredness and to-do list aside to go fishing, I was often grumpy, generating a fresh wave of guilt. During one fishing trip, I asked John if he was having a good time.

"Kinda," he said, "but I wish you weren't so unhappy."

No matter what I did or didn't do, I was always in the wrong, and my debt to the world was becoming a mountain I could never move. One day as I walked to the OAMH Clinic to meet with my support group, I thought about a fellow-caregiver who had been at an event that John and I had attended the previous evening, and a wave of guilt washed over me because I had not talked with this person. In short order, I escalated an unintended oversight (which the person probably never even noticed) into a major transgression. To counteract my guilt, I tried to think of ways to make amends. I could, I thought, arrange a tea date with this person, but my calendar was already full for the coming weeks. I was mentally rearranging my schedule to accommodate this new task when I suddenly stopped in my tracks and gave my head a shake. "Sure, Rosella," I chided myself out loud, "make this happen. And while you're at it, how about knocking on every door in this town to find someone who is a little sad that you can cheer up?" I couldn't help but laugh, and in the laughing, my anxiety vanished—for the moment.

Ensuring that John could continue to fish was a task that grew increasingly difficult—and dangerous—as he transitioned to the middle stage of dementia. Bit by bit, I took on the major tasks that came with a fishing trip—making sure the boat was gassed and ready; hauling full gas cans, rods, life jackets, lunch, water, extra clothing, and sundry items to the boat; and battling with John when he insisted that he could handle the wheelbarrow down the steep boat ramp and along the floating dock even though he was constantly in danger of losing his balance. Once we were out on the water, I tried to encourage him to decide where he wanted to fish, but he couldn't seem to make up his mind and was always worrying about the weather changing. In retrospect, I believe he could not remember his favourite fishing spots, and was often confused, certain there used to be a sandy beach where trees now grew to the shoreline, or there had been trees where there was now only grass. By the end of the 2016 fishing season, he was asking me to direct him where to turn into the marina. That September we went on what I suspected might be our final fishing trip.

Last day of fishing. We were on the water by 7:20. I decided that this was my gift to John and to make it meaningful, I would give it without resentment. Thus, I was fully present with him all day. Aware that he might have difficulty making decisions about where to fish, I gave him a chance to choose and when he didn't, I chose the spots for him. The day was beautiful and peaceful, and we caught many fish, although none were very big. He suggested going in earlier, but I encouraged him to stay out there until after 3 p.m., hoping he would catch something big, a last-hurrah kind of thing. That didn't happen, and as we headed home, I felt both relieved that the fishing season is over and guilty for this relief. I worried that one day when it was too late, I would regret that I didn't value these moments more.

The following spring, I wrestled once again about whether to put the boat in the water.

If I agree to put the boat in the water, I wrote, *my writing time will vanish. If I don't put the boat in the water, his hope will vanish. I am torn between my quality of life and his.*

One stressful, frustrating day in mid-March 2017, after reconnecting John's processor for the fifth time, we left for MIM, only to have him fuss with and disconnect the processor once again so I had to pull over to the side of the road and deal with it. After MIM, I had to deal with even more confusion as we drove to Langdale and took the ferry to Horseshoe Bay to pick up our granddaughter. On the ferry ride back, I hid in the bathroom and gave way to tears. "There is no bloody way," I sobbed, "that I'm putting that boat back in the water!"

To compensate, I arranged with a friend to take us to Clowhom in his cabin cruiser. Three times that summer we went on two and three-day excursions to our old haunts. Our friend was also able to borrow vehicles at both Clowhom and at the head of Narrows Inlet and take us for long drives into the back country, something John had loved to do when he was living at Clowhom. He was in heaven during these drives with our friend and preferred them over going fishing. But eventually, even those trips grew too difficult. As soon as he was away from home for any length of time, he would grow confused, and behaviours that I had come to accept as normal for him began to wear on our friend. Worrying about him and John was just one responsibility too much, and the next time a trip was offered, I begged off, finally admitting that our fishing days were over and another door to John's former life had firmly closed. While John rarely spoke—or I believe even thought— about fishing after that, I could not stop feeling guilty for closing that door, knowing I would be closing many others as our journey through dementia continued.

BUSYNESS

The *shoulds* are rising.
Each one satisfied
Spawns a dozen more.
Expectations build.
I am the one and only,
The all-mighty,
Saving the world
One *should* at a time.
What happens
Should I let go?
Does the world collapse?
Am I forever damned?
Will my name be broadcast
In neon lights of shame?
Or will the unmet *shoulds*
Slowly evaporate
Into a neversphere
Leaving me in peace?
Perhaps it is worth a try.

CHAPTER NINE

Strategies For Dealing With Guilt

INSOMNIA

Lying in bed,
Stomach churning,
Thoughts whirling,
Panic creeping,
Wondering,
Is it something I've done?
Or said?
Or didn't say?
Or didn't do?
Or is it just
Mental indigestion?

I won't say that I ever conquered guilt, but, thanks to my therapist, online assistance, and my support group, I did develop some strategies and insights that helped reduce its impact on the emotional overload I was already carrying.

As children, we are taught to be anxious, afraid, and guilty as ways of protecting ourselves from the dangers every creature on this planet faces daily. These are useful strategies when confronting lions and tigers and bears, or are at risk of being kicked out of the clan, but a bit of a nuisance when we want to say no to someone whose only threat to us is their disappointment, disapproval, or rejection. It is disastrous to a caregiver who is dealing with a constant barrage of demands and must say no many times every day. These emotions are so powerful that books on how to cope with anxiety and guilt have become bestsellers, and online videos on the subject are swamped with "likes."

When I was eighteen, I pasted a passage from *Hamlet* on my bedroom wall: "This above all: to thine own self be true." In those days, the words reflected my youthful values, but as a caregiver, the passage took on an even greater meaning.

The late Manuel J. Smith in his book, *When I Say No, I Feel Guilty*, advocated that as individuals we are the "ultimate judge of all that we are and all that we do."[15] He listed twenty "assertive rights" that each of us has, among them changing our minds, making mistakes, acknowledging that we don't have all the answers and saying no, and he maintained that by taking responsibility for our own actions, we disable the power of others to manipulate our behaviour. His lessons on how to assert these rights, included clearly identifying what we want and then repeating that message over and over. When faced with criticisms levelled against us, we should let go of our initial emotional response, identify the actual error or fault and then, without apology, agree with the critic. This lesson came in handy when a relative commented sarcastically that I was making all of John's decisions for him, including ordering what he would eat in a restaurant. My immediate response was to feel guilty, embarrassed, and ashamed. Instead, I pushed those old reactions aside and acknowledged the truth in what the person was saying.

"Yes," I agreed, "I am making his decisions for him, and I hate it. I would love it if he could make choices for himself." A simple statement, but it left the relative with nothing more to say on the subject and me free of guilt, even if only for a moment.

Questioning the reality of my thoughts also helped me to cope with caregiver guilt and sometimes that meant expanding the original thought. When John asked, "Please sleep with me tonight," I felt guilty for saying no. Then I thought, *Day by day things are being taken from John—driving, fishing, sleeping with me,* and this time, instead of holding onto that thought, I expanded it to: *Every day, things are also being taken away from me—writing opportunities, visits with our granddaughter, travel. It is a two-way street and looking after my health is best for both of us. Without proper sleep, my health deteriorates.* I won't say that doing this eliminated my guilt feelings entirely, but it did reduce them, and I discovered that the more I challenged my perceptions the easier it became to shift the blame for John's sadness or disappointment to where it belonged—a disease that I hadn't caused, could not cure, and certainly could not control.

"There are two ways of viewing what is happening in our lives," my therapist told me. "One is objective, [based on facts that are quantifiable and measurable], the other is subjective [based on emotions and beliefs that are open to interpretation.]" The subjective path, he maintained, has no end. It reminded me of the old Dragnet television series in which the police sergeant always insisted on, "Just the facts, Ma'am."

My therapist also said, "We are never going to get things right one hundred percent of the time. No matter what we do, there are times when hurting happens."

His advice, when I was feeling especially guilty, was to also consider my intent for whatever transgression I had committed or duty I had failed to fulfill.

"Did you *mean* to cause harm? If your intention was pure, don't worry about it. If it wasn't pure, tell yourself you could have done better, apologize and, if possible, make amends. Learn from the mistake and walk away."

The way we talk to and about ourselves also matters. In a TEDx talk, Dr. Kristin Neff says, "…we are often harsher and more cruel to ourselves in the language we use. We say things to ourselves we would never say to someone we cared about. We say things to ourselves that we probably even wouldn't say even to someone we didn't like very much."[16] Her website, www.compassion.org, provides insights and exercises to help people develop mindful self-compassion, which, "combines the skills of mindfulness and self-compassion, providing a powerful tool for emotional resilience."[17]

In my experience, caregivers of persons with dementia need to develop a strong emotional resilience if they are going to make it through the journey.

"I'm giving you a prescription," my therapist told me after one particularly gruelling session in which I poured out a month's worth of guilt and self-condemnation. "For one month go with the emotions that are true to you. During this time monitor John's response. Does he talk about it? If so, what does he say?" It was a tough assignment, but valuable. I began to understand that nothing that I said or did had a lasting effect on John, and that while I *was* responsible for helping him with tasks he could no longer perform for himself, it was not my job to make the world perfect for him.

From the moment we are born until we take our last breath, each of us has our own personal mountain to climb. No one can climb it for us, and we can't climb another person's mountain. Their own abilities and strengths will get them to the peak, or they will anchor themselves to whatever spot they find safest. We can shout encouragement, tell them we love them, even toss them an aide package and hope it lands in a place they can reach, but if we stretch ourselves beyond our ability to hold on, we fall off our own mountain and do no one any good at all.

When I respected the strengths that John and other members of my family were demonstrating, I could trust that I was not as vital to their happiness or existence as I had imagined I was. In fact, by backing off, I let them know I believed in them. In caregiving, letting go happens when we allow others to take over the job now and then.

It is one thing, however, to read or hear about letting go, practising self-compassion, listening, and taking care of your own needs and happiness. It is quite another to insert such ideals into our lives when we are faced with the non-stop demands of caring for someone with an aging adult body and the mind and emotions of a five-year-old. As a caregiver, I often held on too long, and I failed many times to treat myself with compassion. Creating those new neural pathways by learning a different way of thinking and looking after yourself takes time and practice. It doesn't happen overnight, but it *can* happen if we do the work. I know because, in the end, it happened for me.

THE PATH

I was following an old and trusted path
That was keeping me in a place of pain,
Until a teacher showed me how
To forge a passageway not rutted
With false beliefs nor hardened by a past
I could not change.
Unchecked by fallacies, I stumbled forth,
Falling and rising and often losing faith
Until my trembling steps grew firm,
The new trail more defined,
And my guilt dissolved in a lightness of spirit
That drew a smile to my lips.
I was home.

CHAPTER TEN

Advancing Dementia/ Respite/ADP

COMMUNICATION

I want to talk with you again,
To share thoughts.
I want you to know
What I am feeling,
Why I am afraid
Or angry
Or sad.

I want to be heard,
And to hear.
I crave understanding
And empathy,
Laughter,
Even annoyance
If that's what it takes.

See ME, I say,
Feel my pain, I say,
Smile at my whimsy,
Understand that I'm
A little overwhelmed
And give me a hug
That tells me I am not all alone.

But my pleading words,
My baring of heart and soul,
Falls into the abyss
Of your confusion,
And you ask
"Can you look at my knee?
It's hurting."

It never fails to astonish me how quickly the human brain "normalizes" something that is not at all normal. People in war zones and refugee camps and in the aftermath of great disasters adapt to the changes, and the new "normal" becomes so familiar that the old normal is almost forgotten. I thought, because I knew this, that my habit of normalizing John's behaviour might shift as his dementia increased. Instead, I adapted to each change in his cognition so effectively that I could not understand why I was always so drained of energy, so short of temper, and so close to tears. This inability to accept his deterioration was even harder during John's moments of clarity, as occurred one day when we were coming out of the grocery store. On reaching our car, I could not unlock the trunk to load the groceries we'd purchased.

"This isn't our car," John said quietly. "Our number is 060."

I looked down at the licence plate and he was right. I'd gone to the wrong car.

Afraid that I was exaggerating his dementia symptoms, I eagerly accepted Kathy Thomas's offer to reassess John. During the test, his wit was as sharp as ever, and when she asked him what day it was, he said, "The day after the one that just passed." I was sure this meant that his cognitive abilities had not deteriorated, but the test result told a different story.

"John scored eight out of thirty," Kathy said. "Normally, people with that score are in nursing homes."

As dismayed as I was by the result, it was also oddly comforting to know there was a reason for my stress. Soon after, I gave up even pretending to share a bedroom with John and began staying in my own room even when I heard him get up in the night.

It wasn't long, however, before I was back to blaming my high stress levels on my inadequacies and not on John's dementia.

One weekend in early February 2018, just a month after Kathy's assessment, John developed a rectal bleed. The medical clinic was closed, and suspecting that the bleeding was caused by hemorrhoids, I elected to monitor it but not take him to Emergency where he would experience a long wait and exposure to any viruses floating around the community. (This was in pre-COVID days when masking and sanitizing were not mandatory.) The Health Line nurse I spoke with on the phone agreed with this choice. The next morning I woke in the early hours to John thumping on the bedroom wall. He was desperate and afraid—for good reason, I discovered, after following him downstairs to the bathroom. The blood in the toilet was dark and plentiful.

An hour later we were in the Emergency ward where a rectal exam showed the cause of John's bleeding was not hemorrhoids but some internal anomaly. Already castigating myself for not seeking medical help immediately, I was further dismayed when the doctor asked how extensively I wanted them to investigate the bleeding and whether I wanted a DNR notice to be placed on his chart. Years earlier, when John and I had both signed DNR forms, it had been an abstract choice. Now suddenly it was a very real choice that I was not prepared to make.

"I want to know what is wrong," I said at last. "And I need to think about the DNR."

In the end I decided not to put the note on his chart.

I'm not sure if this is the wrong decision, I wrote in my journal, *but I am gambling that it won't be necessary.* Still, it was a warning, and I knew that once this crisis was over, I had some serious thinking to do—and not just about the DNR order.

For three days I dealt with John in the hospital and discovered that this was much, much worse than caring for him at home. He needed help going to and from the bathroom, and when he saw that the bleeding had not stopped, he needed reassurance that it was being investigated, not ignored. Eventually he was transferred from the bed in Emergency to a room on a ward, but that left him even more confused. He thought he was in a very strange hotel and was convinced that I was planning to leave him there forever. On the second day I did escape for an hour but came back to a disaster.

John was in a real state, I wrote later. *He had his jeans out and was getting ready to leave. He was angry and agitated and it took a long time to calm him down, to convince him that I wasn't leaving him, and that he wasn't there on a permanent basis.*

His new obsession with his bowel movements was testing my patience, and I tried to distract him by asking about the biggest fish he ever caught. A long, involved tale emerged that I'd already heard many times over, but as soon as it was finished, he was back to talking about poop.

When I am condemning myself for all the things I did not do for John, I noted in my journal, *I must remember these moments of patience, of listening and repeating instructions and reassurances again and again and again. And that I've made him laugh many times—real belly laughs.*

A colonoscopy revealed that the bleeding originated from a place higher up John's colon than expected. The doctor said it might take surgical intervention to stop it, and the anaesthesia required for the surgery would very likely increase John's dementia. Without the surgery, the bleeding could stop on its own, continue indefinitely with no appreciable difference, or result in a massive bleed that would take his life.

I don't know how much of this John understood, but he said emphatically that he did not want surgery, and I was faced with honouring both this decision and the instructions in the representation agreement he'd signed when his cognitive abilities were still intact. After much deliberation, I said that although I would like to know the cause of the bleeding, the decision was not about me. John did not want surgery, so there was no point in further testing. I was comforted when John's doctor said he would have made the same decision.

It doesn't give me "permission," I wrote, *but it does ease the doubt about whether I am making the right or wrong choice.*

John was discharged that afternoon and was ecstatic to be back home and in his own bed. I, on the other hand, was weeping from physical and emotional exhaustion.

Within a few days, John's bleeding stopped of its own accord, but whenever he had a bowel movement, he would leave squares of poo-covered toilet paper on the bathroom sink for me to inspect. Gradually, he began folding them and putting them in the wastebasket, but he would never again flush them down the toilet. And this, too, soon became normal.

After John's assessment in January, Kathy had urged me to enrol him in the Memory Club held at the local Older Adult Mental Health Clinic. The two-hour program for persons with dementia included exercises, socializing, and a simple activity. It was intended to stimulate cognitive function and to give caregivers a short break to attend appointments, go shopping, or just rest. At first John resisted, but I was finally able to persuade him to give it a try, and when he saw that some of the people from our Minds in Motion group were there, he agreed to go again. Over time, it became part of our weekly routine, providing me with some badly needed respite. I would take my computer to the Starbucks across the street from the clinic and for two hours lose myself in writing. Sometimes another caregiver or two would stop by, and we'd have an impromptu support group that was always uplifting. For the most part, John enjoyed the two hours, but he often grumbled about it on the way home. "Those people are very strange," he said one day. "They cheat at the games."

Despite the Memory Club, my own ongoing mental health therapy, and the occasional respite breaks I was able to take thanks to Patti looking after John, my stress levels continued to rise as John's dementia grew steadily worse. Now, I was not only feeling as if I was in prison, but also as if my prison cell was shrinking with every passing day. Through the bars I could see life going on without me. My oldest brother, who lived some distance away, was diagnosed with terminal cancer, but I was unable to visit him because I didn't want to leave John. My granddaughter was growing up, and I was missing opportunities to be with her. I had no time to spend with my friends or to attend events that would help my writing career. As a result, love gradually gave way to resentment and frustration, and when these feelings overflowed in the form of angry words or slammed doors, guilt took their place.

One morning in May I woke to John calling frantically from his room. I hurried to his side and was horrified to find that his right eye was filled with blood. A window in his room looked out onto the municipal works yard where the workers would often arrive before daylight, their headlights shining through the bedroom window as they turned into the works yard. John was convinced that one of these workers had deliberately directed a laser beam at him, damaging his eye. That afternoon I took him to the eye clinic where an ophthalmologist assured him that the hemorrhage was not caused by a laser beam. No exact cause for the bleed was determined, and it eventually cleared with no harm done to John's vision. His fixation on the laser attack, however, remained. From then on, he kept the blind down on the window and told the story of the laser attack over and over to me and anyone else who would listen. What made it worse was his anger. One night after looking at his eye in the mirror, he snarled, "If I see those sons-of-bitches doing that again, I'm going to get out my gun and shoot them!"

Soon after this, he became convinced that our house was a boat, and every night he would fuss about it not being anchored properly. His discontent was hard to take.

I am giving up so much to keep him happy, I wrote, *and it is like I am doing it for nothing. He might as well be in a home. But then he tells me how grateful he is for all that I do, and how scared he is that he might have to go away, and I can't bear to think of doing anything other than what I'm doing.*

My therapist told me that I was not responsible for John's happiness, only for his care, but it was hard to let go of that illusion of control.

Tonight, as he held me close, I realized that so long as those arms are around me, I can pretend that everything is like it used to be, that the world is safe, and I'm loved and protected. But when he, or I, step back, reality returns.

Nor did it help when one day, after I said that I loved him, John replied, "Without you, there would be no me."

At a support group meeting, I tearfully expressed my frustration and despair.

"You need to put John in Adult Day Care," Kathy said bluntly.

I was familiar with the four-hour Adult Day Program (ADP) that had been created to help persons with dementia. It was held at Shorncliffe Village Care Home, not far from our house, but until now I'd fought against sending John there, partly because doing so seemed as if I was giving up on him, and partly because I suspected that with his difficulty hearing he would be isolated in a group situation. John was not keen on the idea either. "What am I doing wrong?" he asked, as if ADP was a punishment.

"Did you ever consider," my therapist asked gently, "that you might be harming John more by keeping him at home? That you might be denying him the social stimulation he needs?"

In the face of such arguments and Kathy's persistence, I finally made a call that put John on the ADP waiting list. *I can always take him off the list,* I told myself, and with Kathy's help I applied to Vancouver Coastal Health for a case manager for John. After a thorough assessment, she approved him for ADP one day a week. A few days later John and I met with the ADP coordinator and had a short tour of Shorncliffe.

"Being in a place like that is not living," John said later, then waved his arm helplessly at our backyard. "This is my place. The yard and the work I do."

That evening I went over the benefits of the program with him again and again, trying to reassure him that it would only be four hours one day a week, but he remained convinced that he would have to move there.

I do hate, hate, hate, hate, hate this! I typed later, almost breaking the keys because I was pressing them so hard. *I feel sad and very tired. Not sure if this is the right thing to do. I am doing it because of his increasing confusion and what they say are "hallucinations and delusions"—talking about people who aren't here, about things missing that aren't missing. I am afraid it is a precursor to more severe symptoms, and it is better for him to become familiar with Shorncliffe. But oh, it is a horrible choice. I feel like an executioner.*

In my imagination, I created a place that was so awful that I seriously considered taking John off the list, but before I could do so, I was hospitalized for two days with pneumonia and exhaustion. When I returned home, I knew I had no choice.

I attended the first session with him and was not reassured. Everyone was friendly and kind, but as I had suspected, it was a one-size-fits-all program that met few of John's needs. It required him to sit in one place for four hours, and he was lost when it came to the discussions because he could not hear anything being said. One game was completely over his head, though a bingo game had better results. When we got back home, he said emphatically that he was never going back.

"John," I said, taking his hand, "I don't like it, and you don't like it, but it is what we must do so you can stay at home, and for me that makes it worth doing."

In the end, although he agreed to attend for my sake, he continued to resist going and for the first few months I had to pick him up early from the program because he was becoming agitated and wanted to go home. Still, I persisted and eventually, as the doctors and Kathy and the staff at Shorncliffe promised, ADP became a part of our routine, one that John accepted and sometimes even enjoyed, especially when I was able to take him for a drive and a walk before the program.

I would like to say that one day a week at the ADP solved my stress issues, but it didn't. After a while, I added more ADP days and hired a care aide to take him for walks three times a week. On ADP days, she would pick him up at Shorncliffe, giving me six hours to myself. Yet even that was not enough.

You're being selfish! I berated myself. *The more time you get, the more you want!*

Self-blame was easier to bear than the reality that John's dementia symptoms were increasing and even affecting his eating habits. It is common for persons with dementia to have difficulties recognizing familiar foods and with chewing and swallowing. The man I married loved blackened toast, the tougher the better, but this stranger who was occupying his body wanted it lightly toasted and the crusts removed. He began avoiding anything that had to be chewed and became sensitive to colour, shape, and texture, refusing to eat foods such as rice and stir-fries. Although he still ate meat, he did so grudgingly and insisted it be ground or cut into small pieces. His clothing choices were also shifting, and it was now necessary for me to lay out his clothes in the morning. If I didn't, he'd come down in something inappropriate, such as one of my own shirts, and complain that it no longer fit properly. Speaking also became increasingly difficult for him. His voice became so soft I could hardly hear him, and he struggled constantly to find the words he needed to say what he wanted to say.

And yet, there were still windows of startling clarity. One morning, he looked out at the sky and said, "It has a blue skin and no clouds." Another time, when I remarked that time was going too fast, he grimaced and said, "For me time has stopped."

Without wanting to, I felt myself withdrawing from him more and more, and I often wondered, *Am I withdrawing from him because his condition is deteriorating, or is his condition deteriorating because I am withdrawing from him?* Between the grief I was constantly feeling as I watched him slowly slip away from me and the stress building from being on-duty night and day, I began to doubt my own sanity.

One of John's changing behaviours was his declining interest in reading or watching television, two activities that I relied on to keep him in one place for a short time. One cause of this change was the cataracts he'd developed in both eyes. His ophthalmologist had warned that if he did not have cataract surgery now, when he could still provide the responses required to test his vision, it would be too late. She suggested operating on one eye first and the second a month later. The thought of him not being able to see combined with his hearing disability was more than enough to motivate me to agree to this, even though it meant more trips to the city. Fortunately, my sister opened her home to us, and we were able to stay in town the night before his first surgery.

We presented at the Eye Care Centre early in the morning. John was duly gowned, prepped, and taken into the surgical ward, but partway through the surgery, the nurse motioned to me to come in as well. Somehow, John's processor had become disconnected, and he could not hear the surgeon's instructions to look in the direction that would enable her to access his retina. I was gowned, masked, and gloved and directed to the OR table, but there was no way I could reconnect the processor without moving John's head. Instead, I took his hand and by moving it in the required direction managed to get him to look that way. I could watch the surgeon's deft moves on the monitor above John's head, a fascinating show had it not been for the realization that if he didn't keep his eyes turned in the direction needed, his ability to see would be severely compromised. By the time the surgery was finished, my arm was aching and stiff, but the new lens was safely installed and secured. We left the Centre with eye medication and stern instructions for John to keep the eye patch in place and under no circumstances to scratch his itchy eyes. Right.

That night I slept very little, fearing every time John moved that he was about to touch his eye. The surgery improved John's vision, but we never did go back for the second operation.

It seems to be a human condition to want our efforts to be recognized. As John's needs increased, my need to have things I was doing for him valued also escalated, and it became harder and harder for me to tolerate his disbelief that anything was wrong with him.

It minimizes the sacrifices I'm making, I wrote after listening to him insist that he could look after himself. *I don't expect thanks or endless gratitude. I just want my efforts to be validated.*

Although I was prone to questioning my own assessment of John's dementia, it bothered me when someone who had not seen him in a while commented that he seemed perfectly normal. At my support groups I had learned about denial—the inability to accept that someone you love has dementia. Rather than looking for signs that tell them the disease exists, relatives and friends fixate on signs that says it does not. Knowing this helped me to understand the why, but it did not lessen the hurt or frustration when my caregiving difficulties were not acknowledged.

It is not just the duties of caregiving that are stressful, but the life events that occur naturally in everybody's life. Normally we take these mishaps or disasters as they come, deal with the grief, pain, or discomfort and move on. But when a person has already used up their reserves of emotional or physical abundance, a simple mishap can become catastrophic. Thus, when a rat had invaded our home, I came dangerously close to hysteria. Night after night until the saints that operate our local pest control company took care of the problem, I would lie awake fearfully analyzing every sound our creaky old house made. Never again did our home feel completely safe to me.

I was so beaten down by the rodents, by John's needs, and by my duties as a mother, grandmother, writer, and landlord, that when I went to the hospital for a colonoscopy—an uncomfortable procedure dreaded by most—I felt as if I was having a spa day. The bed was comfortable, caring staff brought me warm blankies, and I had nothing to do but wait for the medics to do their thing. It was a treat I didn't want to end.

Sometimes my worries became so overwhelming that I blanked out.

I couldn't seem to move, I wrote. *I knew what needed doing, I just couldn't motivate myself to move.*

In the midst of all these other issues, my vacillation about having sex with John continued to generate guilt, grief, anger, and resentment. I wrote often in my journal as I struggled to find a solution that was kind to John and worked for me.

The man I loved and married, and the man I feel I am turning my back on now, are two different people. I don't feel the same about him emotionally or sexually because that "John" is gone. This man is a stranger, not my lover, not my friend, not my confidant. And I do love him still, but it is a different kind of love.

When I spoke to my therapist about this, he suggested I consider that no court in this land would find me guilty of anything for not having sex when I didn't want to. He also gave me a prescription: no sex for one month. The relief I felt during that time was intense, but when the month was over, I found myself giving in to John's request, even though intercourse was now physically as well as emotionally painful.

On New Year's Eve 2018, I wrote, *John truly wanted sex, but I said no. I do not feel good about it, but I don't want the pain and I don't want that kind of intimacy with him. And yet I feel bereft from the loss of that same intimacy.*

Although he wasn't quite as articulate, John said that he felt me drifting away from him.

"You are here," he said, "but there is more and more distance."

I had no answer, except that I loved him.

"I know that," he said, "and I love you so much. I think if you were not here, I would just disappear."

In an effort to cope with my guilt, I wrote, *My intention is to love him and myself. I am growing distant because he has receded. His light burns dimmer with each passing day, yet despite that dimming, despite my own physical and emotional needs not being met, I am still here, still trying to make life as good for him as it can be. That must count for something.*

Recording my feelings helped, but it didn't stop me from believing that I was taking one more reason for living away from this man whom I had vowed to love and cherish until death. And it wasn't the last thing I would take from him.

My brother died in mid-December, and the Christmas merriment around me seemed to mock my despair as I dealt with my grief and John's needs. My physical and emotional health declined so dramatically that both my therapist and Kathy urged me to consider long-term care for John. Although I staunchly resisted this solution, after another bout of diverticulitis, I knew something had to change. Selling John's beloved truck and his boat and using the money to provide home care for him was the only solution I could come up with. I rationalized that the additional help would enable me to keep him home right until the end.

Both the truck and the boat were symbolic of John's life as a free-spirited outdoorsman and fisherman, but that man and those days were gone, something even he seemed to know. It had been many months since he'd driven the truck—partly because he could no longer remember how to use the clutch to start it—and I'm sure it was a constant reminder of this failure. Occasionally he talked of going fishing, but I suspected a part of him knew he was never again going to be able to pilot his boat anywhere. In any case, he readily agreed to the sales, and it was I, not he, who wept when first the truck and then the boat left our yard for the last time. John never asked about them again.

Still, he continued to fear that he would be sent away.

DISCORDANT DESIRES

It seems such a simple thing,
Lying here with you,
Your arms strong and ready,
Yearning to hold me
Yet too gentlemanly to reach out
When encouragement is lacking.
I feel your warmth and I want to oblige
But it is from duty, not desire.
So, I say no and cringe as you look at me
With the eyes of a wounded child
Who hurts but doesn't understand why.
Filled with the shame
Of my hard-hearted stance,
My head pounds with sneers
Of frigid bitches and selfish cows.
And still, the ever stronger me
Whispers that my wants
Are also important and my feelings
Deserve to be respected.
The truth is the heart can't feel
What the heart can't feel
No matter what the head demands.
I love you dearly, my husband,
And I am as bereaved as you
That my body and my heart
No longer beat to the same drum.

CHAPTER ELEVEN

The Dementia Community

LOST PRONOUN

There is a *Me*
And there is an *I*
In dementia,
But there is no *U,*
And there is no *Us.*
Dementia is a mind
Turned inward,
Consciousness shrunk
To a single entity,
And it doesn't matter
How loud you scream
Or how many tears you shed,
The door to *U* is closed
And will never reopen.
Me and *I*
Have left the building
Of *Us.*

When John and I first started this dementia journey, his doctor told me that I was not alone and rattled off the names of local organizations and services designed to help the caregivers of persons with dementia. At the time his words went in one ear and out the other, partly because it was as if he was speaking in a foreign language and partly because my brain was already too busy trying to absorb the potential impact of John's diagnosis on our lives. As a result, I didn't seek out the knowledge about dementia or the help I needed until caring for John began to overwhelm me—not because the information and help wasn't there, but because I didn't know how to access it, and I didn't realize how much it could help.

Many services available to caregivers are not well advertised, and the caregiver needs to do a little research to find them. The local medical clinic, library, town or city hall, mental health offices, provincial ministries (in BC, it's the Ministry of Children and Family Development), community service offices, and local seniors' organizations are good places to start.[1] The Family Caregivers of BC website, https://www.familycaregiversbc.ca/, offers many aids to caregivers, including videos, tip sheets, legal information, and a whole section on caregiver well-being that includes helpful articles such as "Checking on How You Are Feeling," "Coping with those Unexpected Changes," "Creative Goal Setting," and "Preventing Caregiver Burnout."

Another source of help and information, even during the stage where dementia is suspected but not diagnosed, is the Alzheimer Society of Canada based in Toronto but linked to provincial branches, including the Alzheimer Society of BC. There are other Alzheimer groups around the world, such as the Alzheimer's Association (wwe.alz.org) in Chicago, and the Alzheimer's Society in England (www.alzheimers.org.uk). These non-profit organizations are dedicated to research, education, resources, and support for those suffering or caring for someone with not just Alzheimer's disease but other types of dementia, including vascular dementia,

---

1 For a list of resources, see Appendix I.

Lewy body dementia, and mixed dementias. They provide information, videos, and links on their websites for every stage of dementia, as well as for services such as support groups (both online and in person) and the community resources available to caregivers. According to Amelia Gillies, Support and Education Coordinator for the Alzheimer Society of BC, "Anyone is welcome to connect with the Alzheimer Society and our programs at *any* point along their dementia journey. They do not *need* a formal referral from a medical professional to do so."[18] However, a referral is required to access their First Link program, which includes the Minds in Motion program (MIM) discussed in previous chapters.

Physicians are one of the first sources of information and support for a caregiver, but I believe they are often the last we caregivers think to approach. At least, in my case, this was true. I always thought a doctor was someone you went to when you had something physically wrong, such as a bladder or ear infection. To make an appointment simply to discuss the difficulties of looking after John seemed wrong on so many levels, yet when desperation drove me to do just that, I found the doctor more than happy to listen and to make the referrals I required to access the Older Adult Mental Health Clinic (OAMH), support groups, and community resources. Sometimes, just having the doctor acknowledge the enormity of my role as a caregiver was all I needed to get through a few more days or weeks of the insane life I was living.

Across Canada mental health services, including programs for caregivers, are provided by provincial health authorities. For example, the Sunshine Coast, as part of the Vancouver Coastal Health (VCH) authority, offers a variety of services, including three long-term care facilities—the Totem Lodge extended care home and Shornecliffe Intermediate Care Home in Sechelt, and Christianson Village, a complex care facility in Gibsons.

The OAMH and Substance Use Services clinic in Sechelt provides services for both caregivers and persons with dementia, including personal counselling to help caregivers with anxiety and depression. As noted in chapter six, it was through the OAMH clinic that I was referred to a psychiatrist who not only provided me with the support, advice and encouragement I needed to look after John, but also introduced me to cognitive behavioural therapy, which provided me with the tools I needed to cope with the chronic anxiety I had suffered from all my life.

It was also with the help of the OAMH staff that I connected with the VCH Home and Community Care office and John was assigned a case manager who determined the services he was eligible to receive and provided the necessary referrals. Some home and community care services offered by VCH are free of charge, while others include a fee that is based on the income of the person needing support and their spouse, if applicable. While this works for many people, the fact that the care aides change frequently is too confusing for others. In our case, the cost was more than we could afford, and the care aides could not take John for walks because we lived in a high-industrial traffic neighbourhood, and they are not permitted to take the person with dementia in their cars to a quieter area. (My solution was to hire two private care aides who were willing to use their own vehicles to take John to a provincial park for walks.) The health authority also provided a foot care nurse, but again the cost was too high, and I turned instead to a private spa run by a lovely lady who would pamper John's feet for an hour while I went for a walk.

Publicly funded or subsidized home nursing care, adult daycare, and long-term care are also provided by VCH through a referral from the case manager, as is respite care, which enables persons with dementia to be admitted for up to a month to a care home, thus providing the caregiver with some much-needed longer term respite. This service is in such demand, however, that it is necessary to book it far in advance, although in emergency situations, it can be arranged immediately.

Among the resources that sustained me most throughout this dementia journey were support groups. Offered by many of the agencies listed in Appendix I, they were presented on the Sunshine Coast once a month by the Alzheimer Society of BC and every Wednesday afternoon by OAMH. Initially, I had to force myself to attend even though everyone in both groups did their best to make me feel welcome. Over time, however, I learned to trust these people who came from all walks of life and were bonded by the shared tragedy of dementia. At almost every meeting it was stressed that what was said in the room was confidential, which gave us the confidence to express feelings and to talk about our mistakes—and successes—without fearing judgement or humiliation. My journal overflowed with the insights I gained at every meeting.

Hearing the stories of others who are really in crisis puts my own issues in a different perspective. It is not that my issues are not important—but seeing what lies ahead on this journey encourages me to value the good things that I still have and to feel less sorry for myself....Everyone bands together to help each other, one caregiver hauling something in his truck for another, or another caregiver sitting with a person with dementia so that her caregiver could go to an appointment.

Our facilitators often stressed that there is a very good reason why caregivers feel as they do. *It helped me to realize that it is burnout and not feeling sorry for myself that is causing my depression. Kathy pointed out that I have not been away from John for a long time, and I've had a lot of other stresses on top of that. I don't like that I am not strong enough to do this without wobbling, but there it is. Hearing this seemed to validate my struggle and I felt better.*

At other times, I wrote about how everyone encouraged me when I was going through a particularly difficult patch or had a crisis to get through. *Today I spoke of how I dread leaving John when I go away this weekend. The facilitator suggested it is not unlike the feelings the parent of a baby or toddler feels when they have to leave them with someone else. That makes sense and I feel much better....I shared how ashamed I am of my discontent. I cried and felt bad because I was dumping on everyone else, but I could not stop myself. Everyone was supportive, and by the end of the meeting I had figured out a solution that might help. It was a slim straw of hope, and I came away feeling drained but so much calmer.*

There were times, of course, when the meetings were sad, especially when we had to deal with the death of the person one of our members was caring for or of one of our members. *One by one they go down,* I wrote. *Our union as a group is tenuous and short-lived.*

Mostly, however, the meetings were positive and often included information that helped us to understand dementia and how it affects behaviours. *I am beginning to understand that John's stubbornness is not directed at me. It is just his way of navigating his new reality—as if he is walking across a pond on floating platforms, he has to move slowly so he doesn't fall into the water.... I have learned so much about dementia this year, about accepting what is happening and consequently dealing with it much better.*

At times the information was about self-care. *Today we talked about boundaries and grieving and self-care. Kathy adapted some breathing and mindfulness exercises designed for nurses so they could be used by us caregivers.*

One day Kathy wrote on the board, "What loss have you suffered on this journey?" *Everyone had a slightly different list, but the things we had in common were loss of self, loss of a partner to share confidences and cares, loss of dreams—it was a good session.*

On another day, the topic was about strategies for coping with panic attacks—the feeling that the walls are closing in on us and we cannot breathe. *The group consensus was that a drink is sometimes enough to break the panic and get us back to breathing again. Just the simple act of making a cup of tea is a mindfulness tool. Other strategies included crying, screaming into a pillow, running, hitting*

something, sitting in a hot tub, and for those who found it meaning-
ful, praying for strength.

Often, the facilitators provided medical information, especially about the medications we had to administer. They also brought in speakers, such as a lawyer who answered our questions about wills, power of attorney, representation agreements and advance directives, and someone from a home care service to talk about the home care that was available on the Sunshine Coast.

Because our facilitators were closely connected with the three care homes on the Sunshine Coast, they were also able to provide insights to those with loved ones in care.

One of the best parts of our support groups was that we were able to laugh, sometimes at a story or joke that a caregiver told and sometimes at ourselves. I shared how the fact that my sister and I looked and sounded a lot alike often so confused John that one day he asked if I was Number One or Number Two sister. Another time, after someone pointed out that I had a self-comforting habit of rocking gently back and forth, I wondered aloud if that was perhaps why John frequently thought he was on a boat. Often we were able to turn something that had made us angry and frustrated into something hysterically funny. At one meeting I told how John had contemptuously pushed aside a sandwich I'd carefully made for him and how I was so furious that I had grabbed the offending sandwich and squished it into mush. In the telling, my fury and resentment disappeared, and I was able to laugh with the others at the image of smooshed bread and ham squeezing through my fingers.

I was always a better caregiver after attending a support group, as I frequently noted in my journal. *As usual, after sharing at group, I was able to be more patient, kind and affectionate with John tonight, and most of my resentment was gone.*

…I asked myself this morning, "Where is the line between John's needs and my needs?" I arrived at the support group and there on

the board was a list—Ten Duties of a Caregiver. The goal, I learned today, is to prepare a care plan for the person you are looking after. Start with identifying their weaknesses and their strengths and design the plan around these. I felt so much better at the end.

A great deal of advocacy happened during, or resulted from, our support group meetings. The facilitators were often able to guide us through bureaucratic channels to get the help we needed, and we as caregivers found ways to join forces to help ourselves, such as initiating caregiver workshops and creating an alternative for couples who were cut from MIM, which happens when the person being cared for advances to middle or later stage dementia. On the Sunshine Coast, they are transitioned to the Memory Club, an OAMH program which, while invaluable, does not include caregivers. One spring several participants in our MIM family were cut from the program at the same time, and their caregivers suddenly found themselves without a place where they and their person with dementia could socialize together. They were so upset that at the next Alzheimer support group, a group of us caregivers decided to start what we called the Memory Café, a social and activity program for persons with dementia, to run in conjunction with MIM. We rented a space for two hours every week and, mimicking the MIM program, organized some games and social activities and hired a fitness instructor to lead an exercise session.

Through Memory Café, we also arranged group outings, such as picnics at one of our local parks, bus trips to a Christmas concert and lunch in Gibsons and to the Sea to Sky Gondola in Squamish. These were times when the person with dementia felt included in an adventure and the caregiver was able to enjoy some fun and laughter. Eventually, we teamed up with the Senior's Activity Centre, and today from fourteen to twenty-four people attend the program every week, the only requirement being that the person with dementia is accompanied by a friend or caregiver.

Of course, there were times when even a support group could not turn things around for me, and I left feeling as much despair as I had arrived with, but these times were few and were far outweighed by the benefits I received from sharing my burden and helping others with theirs. More than anything, the support groups helped me to understand that I was not alone in a journey that is incredibly lonely.

When talking about the dementia community, I would be greatly remiss if I did not emphasize the importance of family and friends. They helped me to survive as a caregiver and contributed to John's well-being during his journey through dementia. I will never lose my gratitude for the gifts they gave to me of time, encouragement, and assistance in everything from boat trips for John when I could no longer provide them, to yard care, respite opportunities, and, at times, even meals. My therapist once told me when I was worrying about paying back the many, many gifts I was receiving that in doing so I was denying people an opportunity to give for giving's sake. It was good advice because there is no way in my lifetime that I could adequately repay these kind and generous people for their help. What I can do, and shall always strive to do, is acknowledge their generosity and pay it forward in any way I can.

In every community there are many kind, well-intentioned people who care about persons with dementia and are striving to put in place systems of support for them and their caregivers. While much is still needed—the greatest of these being more facilities and staff for long-term care and adult day care programs—I am encouraged by groups that are currently working to raise the bar for dementia support. These efforts, and my own experiences, lead me to believe that while caregiving is a long, hard journey, there is a huge dementia community waiting and willing to help and to make caregivers feel not quite so alone.

TALKING IT THROUGH

We sit in a circle of sorts,
And tell our sad, sordid stories,
Talk of our loneliness and sorrow,
Of feeling inadequate,
Of trying desperately to understand
Words that no longer make sense.
We come to this circle
To comfort a soul in despair,
To make life easier for the one in our care,
And to seek forgiveness
For failing again and again.
We sit and talk of these things
And draw brief comfort from our shared misery,
Return home restored
Then struggle for another week
To survive.

CHAPTER TWELVE
The Path Gets Harder

MILLSTONE

For a while today
You were a millstone
About my neck
Banging and bumping
Against my plans
Weighing me down.
I chafed and swore
And snarled
Almost bit you once,
I was in such a temper.
And then . . .
You went to sleep
And as I looked down
At your dear face
My love crept back
And the millstone
Dropped away.

In March 2019, a few days after the boat was sold, John once again asked me to marry him. As before, he was quite astonished when I told him we were already married, and when I showed him our wedding photos, he smiled and declared that he'd never been happier in his life. It was a brief moment of closeness that disappeared later that evening when he began searching for something that he insisted he needed. He wasn't able to explain what "it" was, and for some reason, perhaps partly because he was creating a mess that I'd eventually have to untangle, watching him rooting through drawers and cupboards infuriated me. None of the ploys I used to distract him from his search worked, not even dinner. He ate a little then went right back to searching and by the time I finally got him to bed, I was angry enough to chew iron and spit nails.

John's distorted reality exasperates me when it should be filling me with compassion, I wrote in my journal. *In this crap journey we truly get down to the raw humanity that runs us.*

Once John was asleep, however, my anger disappeared. A humorous YouTube video was circulating at the time depicting a mother being so frustrated with her children that she wanted to wring their necks, but as soon as they left for school or were in bed and sleeping, her anger vanished, and what she'd seen as aggravating monsters were transformed into sweet, angelic beings. *I feel the same way about John*, I wrote. *I hate him when I feel imprisoned or inconvenienced by his disease, but when he is sleeping, all I remember is how sweet he is and how much I love him. Then I feel so ashamed of my earlier thoughts.*

John's dementia was also increasing his frustration. One morning while he was showering, I escaped to my office to do some writing and was so absorbed in my work that I literally jumped when the door banged open. John glared at me from the entrance. He wasn't wearing his processor, and although he was clearly upset, he couldn't verbalize what was bothering him. When I tried to comfort him, he jerked away from me and stormed downstairs. Collecting his processor, I followed and though it took more time than usual, he managed to put it together so he could hear me. By then, he'd forgotten whatever it was that had made him angry and was ready to start his day, but for me, the fear I'd felt in the face of his anger lingered. Even though I knew my reaction stemmed from violence I'd experienced as a child and not John's brief bit of temper, several days passed before my anxiety subsided.

On a much different day John went with me to take some junk to the landfill, which was situated at the top of a long hill near our home. Beyond the entrance to the landfill was an old, unmaintained logging road that provided a little-used, roughly ten-kilometre alternate route to the small community of Tuwanek and the main road that went past our driveway. As we were leaving the landfill, John looked wistfully at the eagles congregating in the trees and asked if maybe one day we could go further up the road. It was sunny and warm, and thinking this would be a nice treat for him, I turned right instead of left. It had been a while since I'd travelled the backroad, and I didn't realize how dangerous the section of the road around Gray Creek had become until we came upon some "Beware of Avalanche" signs. Finding no safe place to turn around, I gripped the steering wheel and carefully guided the car along a narrow path between boulders and tried not to look at the car-sized rocks barely clinging to the cliff face above us. Not realizing the danger, John was thoroughly enjoying our adventure and chattered happily until I finally grated, "Don't talk to me! I'm praying!" Happily, we made it through the slide area and returned safely home.

If I do nothing more for him, I wrote that night, *at least I can remind myself that for an hour today I gave him a bit of heaven.*

John's episodes of not recognizing me as his wife had now become an almost daily occurrence, and he was often upset, asking again and again when we would be leaving and gathering various items to "take home." He could never tell me where home was, and when I explained that we *were* home, that this is where he lived, he would smile happily and relax. Five minutes later he would once again be getting ready to leave.

I worried that the drugs John was taking might be causing his agitation, but since they also seemed to calm him down, I dismissed my concerns and continued with the regime his doctor had prescribed.

Noting my increasing anxiety, both my therapist and Kathy Thomas suggested that I petition to have John accepted for a third day per week at Shorncliffe. He had grown accustomed to going there, and though at times he was restless and wanted to leave early, at other times he was so engaged he did not want to leave when the care aide I'd hired arrived to take him home. The ADP coordinator assured me that they could handle his restlessness and urged me not to worry.

My sister Vera came to my aid as well and offered to trade places with me for a month. She and her husband would stay with John while I took up residence at her home in Vancouver. It was what everyone said I needed—time away from the stress and anxiety of caregiving—but it was not so easy to accept.

It is as if I am consciously destroying my bond with John, I wrote. *I am trying to keep in mind that this bond has already been destroyed by dementia. The person I will leave with my sister is not the man I married. But damn, this is hard!*

My distress increased John's agitation, and I realized this was partly due to him overhearing me talking with my friends about going away.

Be aware of what you say around a person with dementia, I wrote when I realized how my conversations were affecting John. *They may not seem to be paying attention and may not understand what we say most of the time, but they have a kind of radar that will pick up enough bits of conversation to alarm them, albeit not enough for them to understand the whole picture.*

More than once I was tempted to back out of the deal, but my friends and supporters kept me on track. "Do not attach meaning to something that has no meaning," my therapist had urged me, and I took his advice to heart.

My going away is nothing more than me going to Vancouver for rest and writing. I am not giving up. I am not going away forever. I am re-energizing and nothing more.

Fortunately, the part of me that wanted to survive this caregiving journey was stronger than my misgivings. On May 17, 2019, my sister and her husband arrived, and two days later, after dropping John off at the Day Program, I drove to the ferry, tears blinding my eyes.

It took just one day for those tears to change to awe as I experienced for the first time in many years a melting away of anxiety and dread. I had incredible sleeps and woke smiling and refreshed each morning.

I'm feeling incredibly peaceful, I wrote. *I have been feeling as if I were under siege for a very long time. The more peace I have, the more tension eases from me.*

My sister assured me that John was handling my absence just fine and his humour was still intact. One morning, as she was about to pour coffee into his cup, she realized it was half-full of water. "I'll throw it out for you," she offered, but he shook his head. "No need," he told her. "It's only empty water."

Although I was gone, his routines were unchanged and that helped him to feel safe enough that he often mistook Vera for me, telling her she was the most beautiful woman in the world. Occasionally, he would ask about "that other woman who comes around once in a while."

My time away also gave me a new perspective on my feelings about John and his dementia, and I noted in my journal: *I'm thinking that this will be my grieving time for the husband I've lost. When I go back, there will be a man there who I will care for, and I will try to see him as Vera sees him—a man of humour and strength and courage who has dementia—and not as an embodiment of my loss and sorrow.*

They were brave words, but as my respite days sped past, I began to dread their end.

I am craving this peace as an alcoholic craves spirits, harbouring it to myself and not wanting to share it. So long in coming and so short-lived. I treasure every moment.

When I did return in mid-June, John seemed happy to see me and I, in turn, felt much love for him and had a lot more patience.

Once I was home again, life events, as my therapist calls the daily challenges that arise in every person's life, soon intruded upon my peace, and I was once again trying to care for John and still look after the needs of my family, friends, and community. I was determined to maintain the close relationship I had with my bright, energetic, nine-year-old granddaughter, which meant spending quality time with her. She loved her grandfather dearly, often sitting beside him and reading him stories, which he seemed to enjoy. Still, that youthful energy and the disruption of his routines was also stressful, and I was often torn between satisfying John's needs and hers. He responded to my stress by shadowing me, which only increased my impatience and anger—and then my shame.

I think the kids are confusing him, I wrote during a visit when my granddaughter was accompanied by her twelve-year-old cousin, *and I did not have the patience to let him help me with dinner dishes. He sat at the kitchen table, turned his back to me, then rested his head in his hands. When I finished the dishes, I asked if he wanted to go to bed.*

"Is that what I'm supposed to do?" he asked.

"I don't know," I snapped. "Are you tired?"

"No."

"Then don't go to bed. But I'm going to."

What I didn't note or even recognize was that caring for two youngsters on top of everything else I was doing had also drained me.

Another time, already feeling resentful because I'd agreed to do something for a friend that I didn't want to do but didn't have the heart to refuse, I was in no mood to be shadowed. I tried to counter John's insistence on standing right behind me by suggesting he watch TV while I made dinner. A few minutes later he was back in the kitchen, determined to retell a story I'd heard a thousand times before. Losing control, I yelled things I should have kept to myself and cowed him so badly that he went up to his room. I found him sitting on the bed, totally lost; it took much persuasion to make him feel safe enough to come down to dinner. Because I spent much of the evening holding his hand and assuring him that he was loved, he went to bed happy, while I, on the other hand, lay awake for hours feeling small and mean.

Instead of figuring out ways to eliminate these other stresses from my life and allow myself to focus solely on caregiving, I found myself wanting John to just disappear.

I am stuck in this limbo of having no husband but not being able to move on, I wrote. *I hate that I want to end this. The primitive part of me—the part that leaves the old, the maimed and the diseased behind when the tribe moves on—keeps rising to the top, but it feels so unnatural and wrong. John is happy right now. He has no reason for leaving, and he is afraid whenever he thinks of leaving or dying. And yet, his happiness is attached to my being here.*

Once, after a particularly frustrating day, I wrote, *I am so angry with John for existing, and so afraid of him not existing, and so angry at myself for feeling this way, and so angry at this disease for turning me into someone I don't like very much!*

The thought that I was becoming a person I didn't like frequently came to mind, probably because I was so focussed on my anger and resentment that I couldn't see the things I *was* doing for

John, the times that I restrained myself from reacting or tried so hard to get things right, to fix him something to eat that he'd enjoy, to reassure him that all was well so he would feel safe and loved. All I knew was the constant anger and resentment inside of me, the way I seemed to talk of little else besides caregiving with my friends and family, and the loss of the joy, love, and charity that I liked to think was my nature.

Often adding to my frustration were the well-intended but still irritating suggestions from others for making things better for John.

"There is a badminton group starting up," one friend said. "I think John would love it." She meant well, and I had to bite my tongue not to snap at her.

I resent the offer, I wrote later, *though I know it was made with the kindest of intentions. The horrible truth is, I don't want one more thing that I have to take John to or do with him. He is someone I'm looking after, not someone I want to spend time with. Maybe this means I'm a horrible person, but it is how I feel. I am enduring right now, waiting for this journey to end. He is not a husband, and I am not a wife. He is a needy human, and I am the person providing as many of those needs as I can.*

When someone offered caregivers dementia kits that included games and activities for increasing the cognitive abilities of persons with dementia, I felt the same resentment.

I don't want games to play. I don't want to be a couple. I don't want to pretend any more than I'm already pretending that I am oh so happy that John is here and we're together and isn't this all so fricking glorious!

My resentment turned to outright anger when I came upon a poster urging caregivers to understand how the world looks from the perspective of the person with dementia. It is a good message, and I'm sure it helps many families and friends and caregivers to be more compassionate towards the person with dementia, but for me on that day, it was the last straw.

You think I don't KNOW what John is going through? I wrote. You think it MATTERS when I'm up to my butt in alligators? I do the best I can, and sometimes my best isn't gentle or sensitive or understanding!

At times I tried to counter my anger by feeding the nicer part of myself. This stemmed from a story I'd read on the Internet about a fight between the two wolves inside us—one dark and evil, the other light and good.

I am trying to feed the calm wolf and the patient wolf, I wrote, but Snarly and his gang keep grabbing all the soul food and by the time the others arrive, there is none left.

Another time, desperate to shift my mood, I pleaded in my journal, *Come on, lil' grateful wolf! I have some crumbs for you... that's the way...come closer, my friend. We will make this day all about gratitude.*

It might sound silly, but surprisingly the whimsy helped. It just didn't last, and a few days later I was trying once again to make up for my meanness.

I felt bad for yelling at John and confusing him, so at bedtime I sat beside him and held his hand. By then he had forgotten his annoyance and was happy. When he was asleep, I cried a little because I so miss sleeping with him and holding him and being close.

Going for respite breaks, courtesy of my sister, helped and I always returned with my patience and resilience restored. John was always delighted to have me back, though also a little confused.

"So which sister are you?" he asked one night as we watched TV. "Number one or number two?"

"If number one is your wife, then I am number one," I answered, and he was much relieved.

John's dementia had advanced so much by this time that even he was aware that something wasn't right.

"You know, I cannot make decisions anymore," he told my sister, though not in those words but in a way that enabled her to understand his meaning.

The third time she and Frank were on respite duty, John became convinced that Frank was not to be trusted and began hiding everything from him. It was funny, but also another sign of John's deterioration, and when my sister told me about it, my heart broke a little more.

One night as I lay in bed remembering how it felt to be snuggled against his back and missing his warmth and gentle touch, I wrote, *John is in his room, but I can't go to him without messing up his head. I am filled with sadness and feeling so very much alone.*

In January 2019, to cope with my grief and the continuing loss of my husband, I had started to write a book about his life. It would be, I thought, my last gift to him and a way of giving back in some small measure the life he was so rapidly forgetting. Throughout the spring and summer, I spent hours and hours researching his past, scouring genealogic sites on the Internet; reaching out to his family members for their stories and pictures; digging out old letters, documents, John's own journals, and the stories he'd written down; and then ransacking our own photo albums. Sometimes, John sat beside me while I worked, and occasionally I would give him a section to read. At first, he was happy to do so and even read some parts out loud, but gradually it became hard for him to pronounce the words, and he had trouble understanding what it was all about. One day, as he looked at a passage that included pictures of his grandparents, he said in what had become his usual garbled fashion, "They're all dead, aren't they?" When I said yes, he set the papers aside and said, "Then there's no point in reading about them."

Working on the book also meant that during my respite times, when I was supposed to be getting away from John, he was still very present in my mind. Still, it was cathartic for me, enabling me to give back some of what dementia—and, by proxy, I—was taking from him on a daily basis. I felt an increasing urgency to finish the book before it was too late for him to appreciate its meaning, and although I did not make it for his ninety-first birthday as I had hoped, a few weeks later I sent *John's Story* off to the printers.

Vera and Frank had just arrived to give me a respite break that late September day when the book finally arrived.

We all sat around the table, I wrote, *and watched as John went through his book. I could tell from his expression of wonder, and by the way he studied every page that he was really delighted with his gift. No matter that he might not remember it tomorrow, for almost an hour he was absorbed by the pictures and memories they brought up. For me, this made the whole thing worth while.*

A few days later, I wrote, *Today I listened to John read out loud from his book. He seems so happy with it. Sometimes he knows it is about him, and sometimes he does not."*

His memory was the same with me. Sometimes he knew who I was, but more and more often now, he did not. One morning he asked me if I knew when Rosella was getting back. On another occasion, he looked at me closely and said, "I think I used to know you." He wasn't being sarcastic, and it occurred to me that just as he, with dementia, was not the man I married, this cranky person caring for him probably had no resemblance to the woman he married.

When his daughter, Lori, came from her home in Portland to celebrate his birthday, John did not recognize her either, but he was happy that she was there—until he began to suspect that she was trying to lure him back to the States.

At bedtime he was very angry, I wrote. *He said he knew what was going on. He thinks Lori and I are in cahoots and planning to send him away.*

One night as I was putting liniment on his leg, John said tearfully, "Please don't leave me! I am getting better. It comes in little bits." As always, I reassured him that I wasn't going anywhere.

Frequently when he asked when we, or he, had to leave, he would say he needed to get to his people.

"I am your people," I told him once, "and you are my people." For a few moments after that, he was okay, but then he asked again, "When am I supposed to leave?"

Occasionally, I could distract him by asking about fishing or by suggesting a snack, but at other times he would persist in asking the same question for hours. Sometimes he asked where our dog was, or whether the kids were upstairs. As the months wore on, he began more and more to lose his ability to put his concerns into words that even I could understand.

When he came back from his walk, I wrote one day, *he clearly wanted to tell me about it, but he could not find the words or remember enough to complete a sentence, so what he said came out in unrelated half sentences. Finally, he just gave up.*

On another afternoon, he came into the kitchen wearing his boots and carrying his shoes. He said he was getting ready to go down south and was leaving the next day. When I asked him why he wanted to go, he said he wanted to see his folks. "I have lots of friends there," he said, "and my mother. That is my home and where I want to spend the rest of my life." Later he told me his mother was dead and launched into a long string of stories that made no sense. Finally, I said he could not go home tomorrow because he didn't have a passport and that we would see about getting one for him on Monday. As I hoped, this enabled him to let go of his plans and they didn't come back—at least, not that day.

One winter morning I woke in the early hours when it was still dark to find the outside door wide open and John missing. My granddaughter was staying with us that night, so I could not search too far afield and after checking the house and the yard I called first the police and then some friends before waking my grand-daughter. Together we walked down our long drive to the main road, but we could not find him. I was close to panic when an hour later my best friend arrived at the same time as the police—they had found John just as he was turning down our drive, heading for the house. He was wearing shoes but carrying his boots, and he told the constable he had gone to check out the water. We lived just a few blocks from Sechelt Inlet, and I still shudder to think of all the disasters that could have happened to him that night.

The following day I purchased padlocks and installed them on the outside doors. Then I had a long conversation with John about the bad things that could happen to him if he went walking on his own. It was dumb move on my part because, as I noted in my journal, *Now he is urging me not to talk loud or "they" will hear me.*

A few days later as I came out of the bathroom after having a shower, I found John standing outside the kitchen door that, because it was daytime, was unlocked.

"What are you doing?" I asked.

John came in and closed the door. "Someone was calling me," he said.

"Well, they got the wrong number," I said and made a mental note to attach the locks the next time I took a shower.

John's hallucinations were not just voices calling to him.

Today, I wrote, *John was washing up in the bathroom. When he came out, he got his shoes and walking poles. He said two men dressed in white had told him he was very smelly. They instructed him to wash, and then they were going to take him somewhere.*

Besides preventing John from wandering, I was also spending more time helping him bathe. Sometimes in the middle of the night, he'd go downstairs and have a shower by himself. At other times, I would have to prompt him to bathe. When that happened, he often couldn't remember how to turn on the faucets, and I'd have to guide him to the washroom, get the shower running, and turn it off when he was finished. After he developed a flaming red rash on his scrotum from not drying the area completely, I added towelling him to the regime.

The care John needed and the constant vigilance required to keep him from wandering or doing something that might cause a fall or some other disaster was stressful, but it paled in comparison to the anxiety I developed over administering his medications.

Years of extensive research have gone into the development of the pharmaceuticals used to treat dementia, and the health-care professionals who prescribe them are doing their best to create a combination that will work for each individual patient, but this is not an easy or instant process. Just as each individual case of dementia is different, so is that person's reaction to the drugs. While one drug—or combination of drugs—might be the perfect solution for one person, the same drug and dosage can trigger adverse reactions ranging from anger to depression to a zombie-like state in another person.

From the very beginning of our dementia journey, after the Donepezil HCL trial had such a negative affect on John, I had resisted giving him antipsychotic or antidepressant medications. It wasn't until late 2018, when he began showing increased signs of agitation and aggression, that I finally agreed to a prescription for Trazedone, a serotonin modulator that is designed to treat depression. My goal at that time was to ease John's suffering, though as his dementia progressed and his restlessness increased, I think my motivation for administering medications had become as much to ease my distress as it was to alleviate his.

John was physically very strong and much bigger than I am, and although he never raised a hand to me, the underlying expectation of violence was always there for me. The constant vigilance required of me to make sure he didn't wander, coping with his endless searching for some thing or place that did not exist, and the sleep deprivation I was experiencing because of his nighttime prowling was exhausting me. And I was afraid to take sleep medication myself in case I failed to wake when he needed me.

At the same time I felt completely unqualified to handle the trial-and-error process of finding the right combination of drugs to reduce John's symptoms. When the medications appeared to work, I was relieved. When they stopped working and the dosage was increased or a new drug was added, resulting in a distressing reaction, I felt as if I was torturing him.

I gave him half a tablet, I wrote after one particularly trying night, *but it took several hours for him to relax and stop wondering where he was and what he was supposed to be doing.* After giving him his medications on another evening, I noted, *John was very confused tonight. Kept asking how long we could stay here, and he didn't know where to sleep.* Sometimes I would try to rationalize the benefits of the medication. *I find myself blaming the pills for John's erratic behaviour, but the truth is that his dementia is increasing.* At other times I chided myself for administering them. *I find myself thinking about the Dementia Village in Langley where it is said there is no sundowning and the patients are not on any medication. I feel as if I am somehow failing.*

As my concerns mounted, I returned to the doctors again and again and spoke to pharmacists and any other health-care professional I could find willing to discuss the issue and always asked the same questions: "Is this drug harming John more than it is helping him?" and "Am I doing it wrong?" The mixed answers I received only served to endorse my conviction that I was not qualified to be administering such powerful medications. *I spoke to the pharmacist about John's medications,* I wrote. *He said they are not the pills John needs during the day. They are meant for nighttime, but any adjustments to the dosage would have to be done by John's doctor. So I did not give John the medication all day. He was not agitated, but he was confused.*

I wasn't reassured when the medication was changed to a new antipsychotic that came with a black box warning from the FDA that for patients with dementia its use could be linked to heart failure causing death. Other side effects included constipation and weight gain.

I had the prescription filled, but I just couldn't bring myself to give it to John tonight. I will have to think about it for a while. It is horrible to have such a decision in my hands. The doctor was super nice and assured me if he were in my position, despite the warnings, he would give the medication to his loved one to provide them with some relief.

Reassurances from other caregivers who were administering the same medication to the person they were caring for and reported that it was helpful did not comfort me, nor did the answers I received from the nurses. *Kathy Thomas said she did not think half a tablet would hurt John,* I wrote. *She said that it might make him more relaxed, and his knee would hurt less.*

Two days after I began giving John that new medication, I noted, *John took all morning to wake properly. He would sit in the chair and sleep, then get up and sit someplace else and sleep again. When I told him we were going out after lunch, he began obsessing about getting ready, and I finally had to stop everything I was doing, get out his clothes and set up the shower for him, even though it was hours too early. After the shower he seemed a bit clearer.*

Twelve days later, I wrote of a violent incident with one of John's friends who had stopped by to visit. *As our friend prepared to go, I gave him a hug. John was standing nearby, and when our friend touched his shoulder briefly, John became really angry. "No!" he said sharply, then started shoving our friend and demanding loudly, "How do you like it? Hmm? I remember you. Always the same!" I managed to insert myself between John and our friend and said, "Stop it!" but I had to repeat the order three times before John backed off. Our friend was stunned. I tried to reassure him that it was dementia, not John, who was talking, but I know his feelings were hurt. It really made me sad. I'm not sure if it is the dementia worsening, or if it is the medication. I feel so muddled and stupid and anxious and uncertain about this. I just don't know what the right thing is to do.*

I worried that my sister, Vera, would not be able to manage him during my next scheduled respite break, but she didn't think it would be a problem. She felt his behaviour had been "off" before he began taking the new medication.

Not knowing what else to do, I continued to give him the drugs, adjusting and readjusting the dosage as the doctors suggested, though torn each time by my endless internal debate: was I helping or harming him? One night he managed to convey through garbled sentences that he was feeling very afraid and could not understand what was wrong with him. *I told him the doctor had given me a pill that might help him feel calmer,* I wrote. *He said he would like to take it, so at 4 pm I gave him half a pill. Before it took effect, I recorded what he was saying, and it was pretty much the same as before. He rambled on and on, but by 4:30 he was not so anxious.*

Sometimes the medications seemed to work just as they were designed to do. *With this new medication,* I wrote one night, *John is laughing again. A happy laugh, not sarcasm. He is still obsessing, still hearing people telling him what to do, but he's happy and that makes it easier to take.* This result was echoed a few weeks later. *I gave John his medication at 3 p.m. and again at bedtime, so he did not have the paranoia tonight that has been so difficult to handle the past three nights. I don't like doping him up, but he seems happier with it and the medication does not appear to alter his cognition. Even if it does, I can't take the paranoia, and I don't think it is pleasant for him either.*

Still, on days when he was especially confused and disoriented, I would blame it on the medication and cut back the dosage, often with drastic consequences. *I did not give John the morning pill,* I wrote. *I wanted to see how he reacted without it. At 4 p.m. he got very hostile. I'm not sure what set him off, but I decided it was a good time to have dinner. He was a little less resentful, but not much. No more cutting back on the medications!*

Instead I went back to the doctor again and again, and he patiently tweaked and re-tweaked the medication and the dosage. The results would vary, sometimes working for a few days, and sometimes not. *Himself slept till 2:30 a.m.,* I wrote. *He had to pee but couldn't walk, so I took a bucket upstairs and that worked. Tonight, I will cut the pill in half so he can walk. At 10 a.m. he was confused, his speech thick and slurred, and he was still having difficulty walking and keeping his eyes open. He was also very cross. I am feeling guilty for having caused this even though I was only following the doctor's instructions. I was desperate for a night's sleep, and I thought John would benefit from the same. I had no way of knowing how the pills—or combination of pills—would affect him, and I was afraid of withdrawal symptoms if I withheld them.*

Administering medications is a giant hurdle for most caregivers, and something that needs to be addressed through training or closer supervision and monitoring by professionals, but it was not this dilemma alone that was pushing me closer and closer to the edge of my endurance. The truth was that John's needs were becoming greater than one person could provide for on her own, but it was not a truth that I could bring myself to accept. And so, the two of us stumbled from one day to the next, sometimes snarling, sometimes yelling, and sometimes just sobbing our hearts out.

As my case worker promised, John's time at the Adult Day Program was increased to three days per week. Since the program lasted from 10 a.m. until 2 p.m., at which time the private care aides I'd hired would pick him up and take him for a walk, this gave me a full six hours of freedom. Combined with the respite breaks that Vera and my friend, Patti, continued to provide, I was managing, although I was still often filled with guilt for taking these breaks.

"John said he felt that no one wanted him around," the day program coordinator told me one day. When that brought me close to tears, she hastened to assure me his feelings were the result of his dementia and not a failing on my part. "It is one thing to be with him for four hours and enjoy him," she insisted, "and quite another to be dealing with him twenty-four-seven."

The coping skills I had learned through my therapy sessions were also helping me to deal with my guilt and shame. *I feel what I feel*, I wrote after one particularly trying day. *It is what I DO that matters, and what I do is go back and try my best and keep my head above water. I balance my mistakes with successes, my moments of weakness with strength and my criticism and judgement with appreciation and applause.* At bedtime, to soothe myself to sleep, I would repeat over and over, "*I am a strong, caring person. I have support all around me, and I will get through this.* Occasionally, however, my self-talk was a bit sterner. *I am no longer shielding John from his disease. No longer trying to be the perfect caregiver. If I'm busy making supper and he's standing around looking lost and undirected, so be it. If I try to be the perfect caregiver, I'm going to end up being a dead caregiver.* And sometimes stealth was my solution. *Today I woke at five*, I wrote. *I heard John get up and go downstairs. At 5:30 I slipped quietly downstairs and heard him having a shower. Sneaking back upstairs, I turned on my computer and was absorbed in checking emails when I heard him returning. Desperate for a few more moments to myself, I hid behind the door until he went into his bedroom. As I hoped, he went back to bed, and I was free! Such is the false life of a caregiver. We smile when we want to scream, say nice words when we want to snarl, and hide like thieves to steal a few moments of solitude.*

That fall, one of my tenants moved out, and her apartment required extensive renovations before it could be leased again. Suddenly, on top of caregiving and everything else, I was faced with the monumental task of cleaning, arranging for plumbers and carpenters, and selecting new flooring, cupboards, and counters. I became an expert at putting IKEA cupboards together and, as they had all along, my family and friends stepped in to lend a hand and moral support, and I managed get the job done without killing myself or John in the process. Eventually I found new renters and breathed easier, but my relief did not last for long as new storm clouds were gathering on the horizon of my life.

THE PEACE THAT COMES WITH RESPITE

Strange this peace that has descended upon my world;
Not the deliriously happy kind
Or the after-meditation kind,
But a cautious letting go of tension,
Where the feeling of being under siege,
Shifts to an emptiness that is randomly filled
With deep sadness and quiet joy,
Each taking turns throughout the day,
Leaving me in quiet wonder
And slightly bewildered.

There is no moving on in this respite world;
It is only a temporary fix—
The troubles will be waiting on my return.
It is an elusive state wherein the moment
Holds everything that matters.
Tears fall, but are not wildly out of control,
Laughter happens, but does not quite reach the soul,
And the mind very wisely does not stray
To worry lanes or shoulda-coulda avenues.
Do Not Disturb signs exist for a reason.

CHAPTER THIRTEEN

The Power Of
A Good Quote

POCKETS OF JOY

I never know from whence they come,
These pockets of joy
That begin somewhere in the chest,
Flow through every cell of my being
And linger in my smile.

Sometimes they arrive when I am driving,
When I glimpse the grey and white surf
As it rises in an angry huff that breaks
And floods the shore with frothy spray
Then gently recedes to huff some more.

Sometimes it is when I am walking
And a mist touches my cheek,
Or a crow scolds me from a high perch,
Or I see a white unbroken plate lying beside the road
Reminding me of stories waiting to be told.

Sometimes it is in the laughter of a child
Or someone being kind or brave or vulnerable.
Occasionally it appears after I have bared my soul
To others, emptying my pain into their buckets
Of caring and understanding.

They come from everywhere these moments
And it doesn't matter why they appear
Nor how long they linger, but only that they are,
And that I am grateful for the fleeting peace
They bring to my life.

It's funny what can get me through a tough day. Sometimes it's sheer grit. Sometimes it is a joke that comes out of the blue and makes me laugh. And sometimes it is a quote that takes my mind away from the narrow scope of my own troubles and opens it to a wider perception. As William Blake put it, *If the doors of perception were cleansed, everything would appear to man as it is, infinite.*

Fortunately, deep thinkers have been sharing their wisdom for centuries, and it is hard to find a situation that can't be matched with the recorded thought of some fellow human who has shared the same experience. They can be found in books, in the words of songs, and online. When I read or hear these quotes, I feel connected to my fellow humans and not quite so alone or hopeless. After all, if others have faced similar difficulties and survived, is there not a good chance that I will do the same?

I turned to history for the following bits of wisdom that I have found inspirational over the years—if only because they shifted my focus away from my troubles for a few moments.

ABSOLUTION was badly needed while I was a caregiver, struggling beneath a mountain of guilt that grew higher and heavier with every harsh emotion I felt and with every mistake and hard decision I made. An apt quote frequently helped me to accept the truth that I am human, that humans are far from perfect and that sincere emotions are as involuntary as breathing.

No one is perfect—that's why pencils have erasers. Anonymous

Every morning we are born again. What we do today is what matters most. Buddha

ACCEPTANCE of whatever was on my plate as a caregiver often enabled me to deal with the anger and frustration of those things that I could not control, and I welcomed any quote that helped me achieve that state of mind.

> *God grant me the serenity to accept the things I cannot change, courage to change the things I can, and the wisdom to know the difference.* Reinhold Niebuhr

> *In three words I can sum up everything I've learned about life. It goes on.* Robert Frost

CHOICE has always symbolized freedom for me, knowing that whether I do or do not do something is up to me. When my therapist pointed out that I could choose not to look after my husband, not to travel this dementia journey with him, I felt as if I'd been given the keys to my prison. I did not choose to leave but realizing that I could was liberating. I was grateful when I read or heard a quote that reminded me of this truth.

> *I am not what happened to me, I am what I choose to become.* Carl Jung

> *Each morning when I open my eyes, I say to myself: I, not events, have the power to make me happy or unhappy today. I can choose which it shall be. Yesterday is dead, tomorrow hasn't arrived yet. I*

have just one day, today, and I'm going to be happy.
Groucho Marx

COMPASSION is a vital part of a caregiver's makeup, and I was always kinder when I was reminded that John's actions were the result of his disease and not his chosen way of behaving. Often it was an apt quote that shifted my perspective from "poor me" to "poor him."

> *There is the great lesson of "Beauty and the Beast,"*
> *that a thing must be loved before it is lovable.* G.
> K. Chesterton

> *No act of kindness, no matter how small, is ever*
> *wasted.* Aesop

COURAGE was needed many times during my caregiving journey, and when fear was nipping close at my heels, I found it helpful to repeat quotations that strengthened my resolve.

> *Courage isn't having the strength to go on – it*
> *is going on when you don't have strength.*
> Napoleon Bonaparte

INVICTUS

Out of the night that covers me
Black as the pit from pole to pole,
I thank whatever gods may be
For my unconquerable soul.
In the fell clutch of circumstance,
I have not winced nor cried aloud.
Under the bludgeonings of chance
My head is bloody, but unbowed.

Beyond this place of wrath and tears
Looms but the Horror of the shade,
And yet the menace of the years
Finds, and shall find, me unafraid.
It matters not how strait the gate,
How charged with punishments the scroll,
I am the master of my fate
I am the captain of my soul.
(William Ernest Henley)

EMPOWERMENT over my doubts helped me leap many hurdles as a caregiver, and I welcomed any tool that increased my confidence, including just the right quote read or heard at just the right time.

> *You see things; you say, "Why?" But I dream things that never were; and I say, "Why not?"* George Bernard Shaw, *Back to Methuselah*

> *When everything seems to be against you, remember that the airplane takes off against the wind, not with it.* Henry Ford

GRATITUDE is often lost in the depression and despair that accompanies caregiving. Finding something to be grateful for at the end of each day was a way to remind myself that there was still light in this world that had become so dark, and it was often a quote that encouraged me to look for that light.

> *Every experience, no matter how bad it seems, holds within it a blessing of some kind. The goal is to find it.* Buddha

There are only two ways to live your life. One is as though nothing is a miracle. The other is as though everything is a miracle. Albert Einstein

HOPE was often lacking in my caregiving journey, especially after John entered the later stages of dementia, and I welcomed any quote that gave me even the slightest bit of optimism.

Keep your face always turned toward the sunshine— and shadows will fall behind you. Walt Whitman

Nothing is forever except change. Buddha

HUMOUR, the ability to see the funny in the insanity and heart-ache that I dealt with as a caregiver, frequently helped me to shift my attitude from that of a victim to a survivor, and I often found that humour in quotes that someone would post on Facebook or send to me in an email.

Be yourself; everyone else is already taken. Oscar Wilde

I have not failed. I've just found 10,000 ways that won't work. Thomas A. Edison

MINDFULNESS was something I knew nothing about before I became a caregiver, but it became one of the most powerful tools in my armoury when I was experiencing the anxiety and discord triggered by John's increasing dementia, and I was grateful for any quote that led me to this state of being.

Do not dwell in the past, do not dream of the future, concentrate the mind on the present moment. Buddha

The question is not what you look at, but what you see. Henry David Thoreau

PERSEVERANCE while I was dealing with exhaustion and despair as a caregiver sometimes meant holding on for just one more day or hour or even just minute, and there were times when repeating a pertinent quote kept me from letting go.

> *I think I can, I think I can, I think I can, I think I can . . . I thought I could . . .* Rev. Chas. S. Wing, "Story of the Engine That Could," *New York Tribune,*1906

> *What does not kill me makes me stronger.* Friedrich Nietzsche, *Twilight of the Idols.*

REASSURANCE came from quotes that helped me to cope with the anxiety that was a constant companion during my caregiving journey.

> *You're braver than you believe, and stronger than you seem, and smarter than you think.* A.A. Milne, *Christopher Robin*

> *Never let the future disturb you. You will meet it, if you have to, with the same weapons of reason which today arm you against the present.* Marcus Aurelius, *Meditations*

SOLACE was something I needed many times as a caregiver, and I often found it in a quote that addressed the grief that I was feeling as my husband slipped farther and farther away from me, taking with him the life I had thought I would live with him.

Rosella M. Leslie

Only people who are capable of loving strongly can also suffer great sorrow, but this same necessity of loving serves to counteract their grief and heals them. Leo Tolstoy

Time is a sort of river of passing events, and strong is its current; no sooner is a thing brought to sight than it is swept by and another takes its place, and this too will be swept away. Marcus Aurelius

STRATEGIES were always welcome when I was caregiving, and so was any quote that helped me to deal with the uncertainties that frequently plagued my days.

Sometimes our light goes out but is blown again into instant flame by encounter with another human being. Albert Schweitzer

Do what you can, with what you have, where you are. Theodore Roosevelt

WORTHINESS, that belief that you have a right to be and that your efforts as a caregiver have merit, was often lacking as I struggled to meet John's ever-increasing needs, and I was grateful for any quote that helped me feel better about what I was doing.

How far that little candle throws his beams! So shines a good deed in a weary world. William Shakespeare, *The Merchant of Venice*

There is no happiness like that of being loved by your fellow creatures, and feeling that your presence is an addition to their comfort. Charlotte Brontë, *Jane Eyre*

I would have ended my life — it was only my art that held me back. Ah, it seemed impossible to leave the world until I had brought forth all that I felt was within me. Ludwig van Beethoven

PERSPECTIVE

If Ludwig van Beethoven had been
The caregiver of a demented soul,
Would we still celebrate his birth
Or delight in the haunting notes
Of *Für Elise?*
If caregiving had dominated
The life and time of Wolfgang Mozart,
Would his *Rondo Alla Turka*
Or *Eine Kleine Nachtmusik*
Not have been writ?

And yet . . .

Beethoven was beaten as a child
And dealt with ever-increasing deafness.
Mozart was often in debt
And suffered from mental illness.
But neither stopped,
Nor fell back upon excuse or blame.
They found a way despite dire circumstance
To release the song within
And in the wake of living left
Their melodies.

CHAPTER FOURTEEN

Surrender

I THINK I'M GOING TO HELL

Always thought I was
A kindly soul,
Standing by my man,
Loving him
Through thick and murky.
Hard to realize
That isn't so;
Hard to accept
The evil within
That wants to let go.
Not enough room on this raft
For both of us;
Someone needs to get off,
And I have no intention
Of leaving.
Not yet.
Not now.

He's had his time,
I tell myself,
Had a good life—
If you don't count the
Beatings as a kid
Or the marriage
That didn't work—
But shit happens to all of us,

Right?

Only this shit,
This stand-by-your-man crap,
Weighs heavy on my guts
And in the end
Might sink me first.
Therein lies the insanity—
Competing with someone
You love
For the only seat
On the boat.

It had been over ten long years since John was first diagnosed with early dementia, and the road was getting rougher. Despite community supports, drugs, stealth strategies and good intentions, self-reproach, panic attacks, and depression were becoming *my* new normal.

Merry fricking Christmas, I wrote at 5 a.m. on December 25, 2019, after enduring another night of sleep interrupted by John going up and down the stairs. There were many reasons for me to feel grateful that day—I'd just had a three-day visit from my granddaughter and the house had been filled with her laughter as we worked on Christmas crafts, baked and decorated gingerbread cookies, and watched old movies, sometimes with John participating, at others with him watching. I had lots of phone calls from caring friends and family and all the things I needed to prepare a salmon feast for John and me for dinner. It *should* have been a joyous time, but I could not shake the depression I was feeling for long enough to do the things that might have encouraged happier feelings. Just the thought of dragging out the tree and boxes of ornaments was too exhausting. Looking back on it, I think John would probably have enjoyed the lights and tinsel, but since he had no awareness that it was Christmas, it didn't seem worth the bother. No one would be visiting, and although one of John's care aides had helped him to purchase a gift to go along with the special picture he made for me at Memory Club, and I had purchased gifts for him, I was in no mood for opening presents. So I treated the occasion as just another day to get through and wallowed in self-pity, hating him, and hating myself even more.

I feel defective more than ashamed, I wrote that night. *As if I should be handling this better. Christmas is about giving and loving, and I am feeling just the opposite. I know I have much to be grateful for, and I am afraid that this self-pitying, selfish, hard-hearted, small-spirited state I am in will destroy all that is good in my life. And still, the anger rises, the rage burns, and the sorrow deepens.*

As always, I was also filled with self-doubt, even about my anxiety. *What if my depression is just an excuse to end this caregiving gig? If I am not stressed, there is no need for John to go into care. Then there will be no writing. No extra time with my granddaughter. No getting on with the life I want to live—as opposed to the life I have been sentenced to live.*

As 2020 dawned and the festivities faded to Christmas Past, I struggled to keep my head above whatever crisis presented itself. One night, exhausted to the point of tears, I wrote, *Life seems to be chipping away at me, piece by piece. I am like John's brain—falling apart one fragment at a time. In any other job when employees get sick or are under the weather, they stop working and go home. They take wellness days and sick days. In my world there is no going home, no stopping work, and sometimes—depending on John's mood—not even a rest break. There is no one who can take my place on a moment's notice, and no way I can walk away from the job of caring for my husband.*

As I noted earlier in my journal, my anger escalated whenever John was shadowing me: *For a while John was whispering because*

133

he didn't want "them" to hear him. "Those guys are carting every-thing away," he said, and I felt threatened by his urgency. I'm sure he was feeling confused and scared, but instead of compassion I snarled, "Who the hell cares?"

But insomnia was my greatest enemy. Even on the odd night when John didn't get up three or four times, needing my attention, I would lie awake worrying about the ever-worsening family crisis tearing at my heart, or about how I was continuously failing my husband. *When I was tucking John in tonight,* I wrote, *he looked at me and said pleadingly, "Won't you please sleep with me for a little while? I won't bother you." How I wanted to say yes! But I knew I would fall asleep and then wake and not be able to get back to sleep. I am just hurting so much, and I know he is, too. But his pain will last only a few minutes. Mine will last much, much longer.*

Fortunately, there were still times that I was able to appreciate the humour of our situation. One day I took John with me to buy groceries. As we went through the checkout, a helpful clerk put our purchases into a bag, which John then put into our cart. Twice I stopped him from including a roll of plastic produce bags that was sitting on the counter. Distracted by the payment process, I didn't realize until I was putting our purchases into the car that the roll of plastic bags was among them. As soon as John was securely belted into the front seat, I ran back to the store and gave the roll to the bemused clerk. "I was sure it was just there," she said, point-ing at the counter.

Worried about my health, my therapist, support group and the health care team working with John all began urging me to put him into long-term care.

"The hard fact is that John will need to go into care at some point," my therapist said after I broke down in tears in his office. "Whether it is now or six years from now, it will be just as hard for you to face. Your brain will figure out reasons why you are to blame, and you will be in the same agony." He assured me that when people go into care because of dementia, they all want to go home, adding that "home" for them is just a word, without any specific meaning. "There is a good chance that the simplicity of the care home will take away some of John's confusion and make him feel safer."

By the end of our session I had agreed to his recommendation that John be assessed for possible admission into a long-term care facility, but on the drive home I was so full of anger and shame that I screamed and screamed and pounded my fists against the steering wheel. How had my plan to care for John until the very end gone so wrong? *There is only one way out of this dilemma,* I wrote that night, *and that is to put John into care, get on with my life and deal with the crap that is going to come from it. There is nothing a therapist or anyone else can do to make this decision easier. I have reached a crossroads where John's path is going one way and mine another. Which one will I follow?*

The next day I decided that there was no way this final step would be good for John. Instead, I listed the reasons why putting him in care would be better for *me*:

1. The prolonged stress is damaging my health.
2. I am getting older and my window of time for being active is shrinking. I made sure John was able to do the things he loved during his seventies and eighties. Now that I am seventy, don't I have the right to give the same gift to myself?
3. I want to write, to be there for my granddaughter, and to connect with my sisters and friends without having to continuously arrange for John's care.
4. I want to do these things while I am still physically and mentally able to do so.

John going into care, I told myself, did not mean I have given up on him or our love. It meant I was investing in my own well-being. We all have a baseline of happiness, and while he might be sad initially after going into care, eventually he would return to his baseline.

Acknowledging that dementia was John's journey, not mine, I began shifting from saying "I am putting John into care" to "This disease is putting John into care." Still, the debate in my head went on and on. *John was up several times in the night,* I wrote a few weeks later. *I could not sleep, and I was lying there thinking of him in a care home and feeling bad about it. At 4:30 I heard him banging and crashing in his room as he was getting dressed. Realizing that there was no hope for further sleep for me, I reversed my feelings. If I could ship him off this morning I would—with a smile. And a happy dance.* But I did not ship him off. I was nice to him. Then a few days later I wrote, *I am thinking that John will be much better off in a care facility where he won't be subjected to my selfishness and rejection. I am ashamed and tired, and I am going to try to do better tomorrow.*

John's own distress was another factor pushing me towards a long-term care solution. He spent night after night feeling confused, alone, and afraid, and during the day he wasn't much better. He continuously said he had to go somewhere, though he never knew where, and he could not understand what he was supposed to be doing. He would walk around the house carrying his coat and his boots, and I had to tell him over and over that we were not going anywhere.

Until this point, whenever he asked if I wanted him to leave, I'd reassure him that I would be with him until death parted us as I'd promised when we married. But after making the decision to place him in care, I began amending that statement. "Even if you go into a home," I told him, "I will still be here and I will see you every day." One day after I said this to him, we hugged and there were tears in his eyes, but he did not say whether he believed me or not.

The assessment tests left John exhausted, and he only scored seven out of thirty. Because of this, as well as his risk for falling and his wandering, Vancouver Coastal Health authorities decreed that he needed to go into long-term care for his own safety. Since he was incapable of grasping what "long-term care" meant, the decision about his care was transferred to me. I said yes.

Tonight, I wrote, *I am scared and sad, but I don't have the weight on my chest that I did this morning.*

As it turned out, the process of getting John not just into a care home, but into a care home that would best meet his needs, was not easy. Years earlier I had been told that if I entered him in the day program at the Shorncliffe Intermediate Care Home, it would be familiar to him when he eventually went into care there. Now I was informed that I would have to take whatever care home had the first vacancy—Totem Lodge or Shornecliffe in Sechelt or Christianson Village in Gibsons, a twenty-three-kilometre drive from our home. However, his risk of wandering meant he needed a secure ward, available only at Shorncliffe or Christianson Village. The caseworker warned me that if I limited the choice to one facility, it would take much longer for John to be admitted. Nevertheless, I opted for Shorncliffe and was told it might be anywhere from a week to a few months before a bed became available. I tried not to think of the fact that a bed would only become available if there was a death on that ward.

As I signed the forms that would start the process, I felt a strange detachment. It was as if someone else was holding the pen. *Tonight,* I wrote later, *although we were at home, John had no idea where he was. He spent over half an hour looking at everything, trying to figure out why his stuff was here. I am wondering if on some level he did understand why the caseworker was here today, and it triggered this confusion. I guess I will never know.*

The following morning my emotions were off the wall—ranging from anxiety to guilt and back to anxiety. Thoughts about how this was my fault were prominent—I gave him too many pills, not enough pills, not the right pills. I hadn't checked his health concerns. To stop this hamster wheel, I repeated the psyche nurse's advice: *listen to the professionals.* And I did a reality check: *John has dementia, and it is only going to get worse. He is going into a care home. If this is a few months, a year or two years sooner than is really necessary, what real difference will that actually make to the quality of his life, especially when compared to the toll it is taking on mine?*

I want to cry and cry and cry, I wrote, *and that is natural. This is the beginning of the end of this very long road we have travelled together. For the first time in 37 years, I will be on my own, and that is a very scary place to be.*

It truly helped a few days later when I took John to the clinic for yet another adjustment to his prescription, and the doctor told me I was marvelous for caring for John as I did. To further reassure myself that I was doing the right thing, I recorded the events of a typical morning in my journal:

> *John came upstairs at 5:50 am. He was dressed and his processor was connected, but he was very upset. He was wearing sweatpants because "someone" had switched his jeans, and they no longer fit him. The four other pairs of jeans I presented had apparently also been switched. Finally he consented to wear one of these pairs of jeans, but only after I promised we'd buy new ones after the day program. Then he objected to the new belt I'd bought for him, and he would not rest until I replaced it with his old belt. By this time, I had very little hair left, but John wasn't done. He complained that someone had stolen his*

boots (which I found hidden under a desk), and he couldn't find his walking sticks (which he'd hidden behind some coats in the closet). After breakfast he emerged from the bathroom with a bag full of facecloths and a roll of toilet paper. I have no idea what he wanted them for, but they accompanied us to the day program where I conveniently forgot them in the car.

John's caseworker said that, because it was going to take so long for John to be admitted to a care home, I qualified for a care aide to come to the house once a week. Between this extra assistance, the day program, Memory Club and help from private care aides, I thought I could manage, and I did—until March 2020 when COVID became a reality that no one could ignore.

At first it was just a matter of wearing masks and staying home when anyone was sick. But after the devastating outbreaks in care homes and the increasing number of COVID cases in the province, programs began to shut down, including the day program at Shorncliffe and the Memory Club at the Older Adult Mental Health clinic. Soon, the Memory Café had to close, too, and I was also forced to cancel the walks John was taking with private care aides. As travel restrictions increased, help from my sister also ended. What was worse was that my granddaughter could no longer visit.

In a strange way my initial reaction to the lockdown was one of relief. *The pressure I feel to visit people and to look after them has been lifted, and I dread this self-isolation ending because everything will go back to the way it was. There is still stress from looking after John, but I think I am handling it better because of the reduction of these other stresses.*

Sadly, those benefits did not last. Caring for John alone, with no relief in sight, was harder than I could ever have imagined.

Here is a John moment, I wrote after one frustrating morning. *He cut the toast he doesn't want into small pieces, his intent being to throw it outside for the birds. Knowing it will feed the rats instead, I told him to put it in the compost bucket. It took many repeated explanations to get him to understand this, but finally he nodded and looked down at his plate. "Someone has cut it all up," he said. I will laugh later. In my jail cell.*

Every morning I would wake from a night of interrupted sleep and be determined to do better, to be kinder and more patient, and to look for the positives in every moment. *This John,* I wrote after a peaceful breakfast, *is the exact opposite to the one I put to bed last night. This John I could tolerate. He is not someone I want to depart from my planet.* An hour later I amended that statement. *That only lasted a few minutes, and then he was on the hamster wheel again, wanting to know where his car was. He insisted that he had to be somewhere and needed to get his things together. This time I asked when he would be leaving, and that stopped the wheel turning. It occurred to me that what he is seeking is a sense of control, and if I don't stop him, he is free to stop himself. We will see. Each solution lasts only as long as it takes for his brain to shift.*

Without the day programs and visits from care aides and friends, John was lonely, and as that loneliness grew, so did his shadowing. One day I was cutting brush on a hillside near the house, removing the old dead plants and making way for the new. Not content to watch from the porch, John started climbing up the bank, which was too steep and unstable for him. I motioned for him to go back, but he either could not understand or would not be dissuaded, and by the time I reached him, he was crawling forward on his hands and knees. It took repeated instructions and exaggerated pantomiming to coax him to turn around and edge himself to a place where he could butt-walk down the bank. I helped him as best I could, afraid with every move that he might roll down the embankment, and by the time he was safely back on level ground, I was out of patience and should have walked away to give myself time to recover. Instead, I began piling the brush I'd cut into the wheelbarrow, and John tried to help by pushing bits along with his walking sticks. I had to bite my lip to keep from screaming at him. That night I wrote, *I am as defeated as I was when I woke this morning. My level of hope is almost rock bottom. I don't see anything changing in time to do me any good. Yet I'm not sure if I were given the opportunity that I would put John into care now, knowing that because of COVID, he would be confined to his room and alone. I may not be offering him much, but I believe it is better than that.*

After several consecutive nights of me getting less and less sleep because of John's nighttime restlessness, I turned once more to giving him pharmaceuticals, which, as always, made me wonder if this was making him worse. His dementia seemed more severe, and I was sure his deterioration was speeding up, but both his doctor and my therapist insisted that the medications he was taking were not the cause. *It is comforting to know this,* I wrote, *but a part of me does wonder if they are just trying to make me feel better. I choose to believe them, since I am not capable of changing things.*

The doctors' moral support did help me to be kinder to John. I began doing word exercises with him and spending time playing a dice game I'd found online. He would become very absorbed in the games, but they required so much concentration that he'd eventually grow tired. "I'll have to be going soon," he'd say, as if he were at one of the day programs. *The purpose of the games is partly to tire him out,* I wrote, *and to make him more amenable to sitting on the couch for a few hours with a blankie on his lap and a gentle nature show on TV. Today it worked.*

As the days wore on, John grew more and more reluctant to go for the walks that had once sustained him. He complained of his knee hurting, said the uneven ground made it worse, and he was terrified whenever we were around cars. Even those moving at a slow speed were going too fast for him. One afternoon he fell off the porch and scraped his knee. Because I'm small and he is not, it was almost impossible for me to help him up, and I worried about what I would do if he had a more serious fall.

A few days later the ADP co-ordinator called to see how we were doing. She said no one was being admitted into long-term care from the outside, only from the hospital, and there was no sign that anything would reopen in terms of respite care or the day program for months and months. I appreciated the update, but the call left me feeling more desperate than ever.

Among the supports I had come to rely upon were the angels who had been cutting John's beard and trimming his nails, two jobs that I could never bring myself to do. I discovered, however, that in a pandemic "never" does not exist, and it wasn't long before I was hauling out scissors and nail clippers. I am still not sure who found this process hardest—John when he saw me approaching with shaking hands and lethal cutting tools, or me as I gritted my teeth and did the best I could.

As in most times of darkness, there were bits of light, and one of the lights in our community were podcasts put together by our local health-care professionals to help people cope with the depression, anxiety, and anger they might have been feeling because of the pandemic. They included mindfulness exercises that lifted me out of my depression, even if it was for just a few hours.

But even the podcasts didn't help with the continuing crisis that was affecting my extended family. Now, as well as John's nighttime wanderings keeping me awake, I was lying in the dark worrying about people I loved but was powerless to help because I couldn't go to them. It was a cry heard throughout the world as the pandemic forced families apart, and reports came daily of a loved one dying alone.

After struggling with insomnia into the wee hours of an April morning, I took some sleep medication, but even that did not bring me the release I needed, and I was still awake at 1:30 when I heard John get up. The sounds he was making were different, and I hastened to his bedroom, entering just as he finished peeing into a basket of winter sweaters and onto the carpeted floor. Too disheartened to even think of cleaning up the mess, I got him back into bed and returned to my room. He was up again at 5:30, and that was the end of my futile attempts to sleep.

In the following days, I reread Viktor Frankl's *Man's Search for Meaning*, and for a while I was able to refocus on finding the good in each day instead of the disastrous. John's doctor called and advised giving John his medication earlier in the evening and to limit his water intake between then and bedtime. Still, my anxiety persisted, and one night I wrote, *It is now 11 p.m. and I should be in bed and sleeping. Instead, I am so full of fear that I don't dare to lie down.*

My solution was to mop floors. Somehow putting my house in order gave me a sense that my life also had some sort of order. As usual, this did not last for long.

I was barely asleep when John got up. At my direction he peed in a bucket, and I took it downstairs then went back to bed. Sometime in the night, he was up again. I heard him shuffling about and making his way downstairs, but I was too defeated to care. I decided that whatever mess he made, I would clean it up in the morning. If he fell down the stairs, well, so be it.

I had suggested several times that he sleep in a bedroom I had prepared for him downstairs, but he adamantly rejected that idea, and the nightly torment continued. After yet another sleepless night, I wrote: *It's 7:00 a.m. and I am sitting at the table with a pain in my chest and a sadness in my heart knowing that I must surrender him to whatever the system has to offer. How much of his current behavior is due to the pills he's taking, I'm not qualified to know. But another part of my family is suffering, and I need to be there for them.*

Having reached what I thought was the end of my endurance, I called the crisis line, but they had no concrete solutions to offer, other than to phone 911 and have paramedics check John out. I couldn't bear the thought of pulling emergency personnel away from helping others in greater need, so I put on my big-girl britches and carried on, spending the rest of the morning talking to my family, walking short distances with John, and weeding my garden while he sat on the porch. For a little while he joined me, getting on his hands and knees and pulling out some weeds. He fell on his teetering way back to the porch, but because of the grass, it was a soft landing. Still, it took forever for me to get him on his feet again.

Exhaustion doesn't cover it, I wrote later. *I'm nauseated and shaking, and I can't seem to talk without crying. John is so incredible. He can barely walk, and he needs help to put on his pants and hobble from the bedroom to the dining room. But after breakfast, he got up from the table and carried his tray to the counter. For the past hour he has been sleeping in his chair at the table. I put a second chair beside him because he keeps leaning to one side.*

I am terrified of nothing changing. I feel frozen in place. I can't engage in anything. My chest is tight, my heart is pounding, and I am so very tired.

Around noon John's doctor called. He said if I brought John to the hospital at 10:00 p.m. he would see that he was admitted, ostensibly to regulate his medications. From there, he would be transferred to long term care. Since there were no beds available in any of the care homes, this meant the hospital ward that had been converted a few years ago to accommodate dementia patients. Since it was intended as a temporary placement, this ward had limited recreational and social opportunities for residents and no access to the outdoors.

"Once John is admitted," the doctor warned gently, "you will no longer be permitted to see him because of COVID regulations, and he will not be able to leave."

As horrifying as that was, I didn't believe I had any choice, and though I cringed inside, I said I would see him there at ten o'clock.

I devoted the rest of the day to doing things John loved. We went for a little walk and had lunch sitting outside. I had told him we would go to the hospital later about his legs and balance, and he seemed okay with that. At one point he looked out at the yard and said, "I don't think I want to come back here. It is all bad now."

At four o'clock, we went for a long drive, and he was happy, urging me to drive further. When we finally returned, we sat on the couch for a long time and he talked and talked, rambling sentences that were not connected to anything I could understand. Then, while he dozed on the couch, I typed up notes for the hospital staff about his medications, his processor, the things he needed help with and liked to eat, and a bit of his history.

We were sitting on the couch once more and hugging when he said softly, "You will be all right." It was as if he understood what was happening and was okay with it. I could barely hold back my tears. By the time I had his bag packed, his notes printed out, and everything ready to go, I was so anxious I had to do deep breathing exercises to keep myself together.

When we got to the hospital, John's knee was hurting so much that he could barely walk, but I found a wheelchair and was able to get him inside. While a nurse registered him and took his blood pressure, his doctor took me aside, and though he reiterated that once John was admitted, there would be no visiting, he also assured me that it was not just time for John to be in care, it was more than time.

The nurse had not been able to get much information from John, but he was taken into Emergency, and I was allowed to come along and helped her get him settled before I was directed back to the waiting room. It was after eleven before I was allowed to return. John was asleep on the bed but woke when I entered. He seemed happy to see me, but he went in and out between knowing and not knowing me, asking one minute if I wanted to climb into bed with him and go to sleep, then asking if Rosella was going to stop by. However, this was probably understandable since I was wearing a mask. He talked and talked, hinting several times that maybe I should go, and finally announced that he was going to close his eyes. I waited until he was sleeping, then kissed him and left.

I felt completely numb as I went out to the car and drove home.

Although my friends and family had called, texted, or emailed their support throughout the day, I had not responded, devoting this quiet last day of my marriage to myself and John.

Tonight, I wrote as I prepared for bed, *I think part of my calm is due to our togetherness today. It has always been the two of us, and crap, I don't know how I'm going to be one of us.*

NO ONE

No one to see my light,
To hear me cry
To wait for my step.
No one creak-creaking
Down the stairs.
No one to hold me,
Arms warm and strong
Heart tender.
No one to take this hurting,
Cut it from my chest.
No one.
Just me.
And this big empty house
Filled with the ghosts
Of us.

CHAPTER FIFTEEN

Tips For Friends And Families Of Caregivers

MORAL SUPPORT

Want you to know how much we appreciate
Your patience in taking our calls,
For listening and helping us along.
We caregivers are a persistent lot,
But our complaints are many.
We get cranky and sometimes explode
And say cruel things, or smash something
Dear to our hearts, to keep from breaking
The one we're looking after.
This is when we most need you to tell us
That we're doing a great job,
Not just once, but every time we see you,
Even if you really think we suck.
Because sometimes the only thing stopping
Our emotions from sliding out of control
Are words of support and praise repeated
Until we start to believe their truth.
Then our burden shrinks,
Our sun shines brighter.
And when the long day glides into night,
We sleep a little sounder.

Before I became a caregiver, I would run in the opposite direction when I heard of someone coping with a family member who had dementia. I was not a bad person or even a particularly selfish person—I was mostly an uninformed person who didn't know how I could make a difference and was afraid of being asked for more help than I could give.

Most caregivers, even when they are close to breaking, will say they are "fine" when someone casually asks how they are doing. This is not a conscious deception—they are usually just too exhausted to describe all the things they are facing at that moment, or they don't want to burden someone who is just asking to be polite, or they know the minute they start to talk about how they are doing they will break down and cry. However, the same questions asked with sincerity and at a time and place when tears can be shed or a long answer can be given can be comforting. One night when I was particularly stressed, I spoke with my son. He asked me how his dad was doing and how I was coping. Two simple questions, but they were asked gently and there was no rush for me to answer, and when the call ended an hour later, I felt as if my son had heard me and that I was loved and not alone.

There are other ways that friends and family members can help without being overwhelmed themselves and without making an unwanted intrusion on the caregiver's life.

One of the simplest ways is to notice what the caregiver is doing and let them know that you are aware of how tough their job is.

Persons suffering from dementia are usually not able to empathize with their caregivers—partly because they don't realize there is anything wrong with their own behaviour. As a result, caregivers often feel as if their efforts are not being noticed or appreciated. For them, "I can't imagine how you are coping without a decent night's sleep," is much more effective and comforting than a blanket statement, such as, "You're doing great!"

For those who can't imagine how they might relate to someone with dementia, it might be helpful to know that the simplest act can be meaningful. Just being present with them, shaking hands, or hugging (should pandemic protocols permit this) is meaningful. I remember John's delighted smile after a friend who managed a local grocery store gave him a hug. He could not hear or understand what our friend said, but he sure knew what a hug meant.

Caregivers are usually filled with doubts and self-criticism about their caregiving, so anything a friend or relative can say to reassure them is helpful, even if it's simply a gentle reminder of the three "Cs"—They didn't *cause* the dementia, can't *cure* the dementia, and can't *control* the dementia.

A good thing *not* to do for caregivers is to give false promises. Don't say you'll be there for the caregiver then blow them off when they ask for help. It usually takes every ounce of a caregiver's courage to make a request, and to have it rejected can often stop them from asking someone else because they lose faith in the sincerity of promises to help. Of course, life events happen, and you can't always be there to honour a pledge, but you can offer an alternative—"I can't help you with this, but I could give you a break for a few hours on Friday." Or, "I can't go to the store for you today, but my friend is going and I could get her to pick up some things for you."

Again, the help you offer does not have to be monumental. It can be something as simple as picking up or returning books to the library or phoning to check in and then listening to what the caregiver has to say or sharing a good joke—laughter being great therapy for a battered soul—or doing some outside work such as raking leaves or collecting and sorting recyclables. Even the smallest task can weigh heavily on a caregiver's shoulders and removing that weight can make the difference between them feeling defeated or encouraged to go on. One friend showed up unexpectedly to take John for a drive. John was delighted and I had a whole afternoon to restore my energies.

It is easy for caregivers to feel as if they are losing their place in the community, especially as the person they are caring for slips into the later stages of dementia and leaving them alone is no longer possible. Reassuring that caregiver that their absence or lack of participation in family or community events is understood gives them the hope that, when their caregiving journey is over, they will still be welcome in whatever social circles they've been forced to leave.

Connecting with friends and other members of the caregiver's family enables helpers to determine what the caregiver needs so they don't duplicate the service that someone else is already providing.

There are many websites devoted to showing friends and families how to help a caregiver, including sites belonging to the Alzheimer Society of Canada, the Mayo Clinic, and the Family Caregivers of BC. Or simply by typing "How to help a caregiver" in your search engine.

When thinking about how to help someone who is looking after a person with dementia or any other illness, remember how even the smallest pebble tossed into a quiet pond can create a great many ripples. Whether it is reassurance, a good joke, or the gift of time or energy, you will make a positive difference in a caregiver's life and quite possibly help them to get through another day of caregiving.

THE BURDEN OF GRATITUDE

Someone gave to me a gift,
And I thought,
I must return the favour
With something of more,
Or at least equal, value.

Someone said it is our task
To honour
The investments in our lives
That are made by those
Who believe we have value.

I put the two together
And realized
Just striving to be the best
I can be will give
My benefactor value.

CHAPTER SIXTEEN

Care Home

CAREHOME VISIT DURING COVID

Eight feet of table, my husband at one end,
  Me at the other, my words muffled
  By the sterile mask covering my face.

He looks at me the way I've seen him look
  A thousand times—a look that says
  This is pure bullshit—and shakes his head.

He doesn't have his glasses, so ignores
  The pictures I have brought and words I've typed
  To show the photo's meaning in his life.

Not understanding COVID or its wrath,
  He rises from his chair and moves my way,
  Arms outstretched and eager for my love.

As I draw back to step beyond his reach.
  I sense that deep within his clouded brain
  He knows that what he's doing breaks the rules.

When I fail to do the same, he looks betrayed,
  And my tear-choked "I love you," is not believed,
  As he in bitter tones says, "Good for you."

He doesn't add that he loves me as well,
  But turns and trudges back into the home
  And leaves me standing outside all alone.

As John gradually settled into the secure confines of Vancouver Coastal Health's long-term care system, our war with dementia shifted. We now found ourselves coping not just with his disease, but with a bureaucracy and lack of resources that meant our struggle was far from over.

Much of this had to do with the pandemic. With so many care home deaths due to COVID outbreaks,[19] the BC government had enacted strict hospital and care home protocols, especially concerning visitors. As a result, and as his doctor had warned, I was not permitted to visit John after he was admitted. For the first few weeks, this was a relief because I was emotionally and physically drained, but as my health returned, so did my need to connect with my husband.

I had been in almost daily contact with the nursing staff on the hospital's dementia care ward, at first because they had trouble with his processor and were unable to communicate with John. However, over the phone I was able to help them understand the written instructions I'd sent with him, and the processor was connected. Then they reported that he was restless and spent a lot of time walking up and down the hallway or heading for the exit, trying to leave, and would not stay in bed at night. Because of this, his medications had been changed to try to get him to sleep better at night. One day when he was insisting that he had to leave, the nurse phoned me and asked if I could speak with him. She hoped it would help settle him, but since he could not hear me, and all I could hear was the distress in his voice, we both ended up frustrated and sad. The next time I was asked to speak with him when he was upset, I refused, knowing it would only make things worse. Fortunately, by the end of the third week, John had settled down and was no longer trying to leave.

I phoned the ward often to check on him, and occasionally, when conditions were just right and he was not upset, John could hear me on a speaker phone. Although he could not understand most of what I said, he seemed to know it was me. Then Zoom calls were introduced, and communication became a little better.

He looked so different, I wrote after our first Zoom call. *They have shaved his beard, and his hair is cut so short he looks bald. He seemed mystified as if he was in a world he didn't quite understand, but he also seemed peaceful. He did not stop looking at me until our time was up. I think for a few moments here and there, he knew who I was and knew I was loving him. I had to fight not to cry, and I so wanted to touch him and hug him. I tried desperately to think of what to say, but few things came to mind.*

As painful as it was to see him in such a remote fashion, it was also comforting to know he was peaceful. I had only to think back on his agitation during the days before he was admitted to appreciate what a blessing that peace of mind was to both of us. Of course, as had happened at home, some days were not so good. He would appear unhappy, defeated, and confused, and I would feel sad, helpless, and guilty because I could do nothing to help him. At other times, he'd remove his processor during the call, or he'd be distracted by something such as a chocolate bar, or would get restless and leave before our time was up.

I find I am steeling myself for these calls, I wrote one night. *Hoping he will look okay. Hoping I'll think of the right things to say. I'm sure he thinks I have abandoned him, which I suppose in a way I have.*

One day the coordinator asked John if he knew who was on the video screen. "Yes!" he said. "That's my wife!" That day he talked more than he had in weeks and said several times how good it was to see me and how he missed me.

It felt as if I had a brief moment with the John that I love, I wrote, *but oh it hurt afterwards because of the memories it provoked.*

One of the benefits of Zoom calls was that his children could join in, and while he did not recognize them, they were able to see how well he was doing.

In July John was finally transferred from the hospital to Totem Lodge. There, he had more freedom to move around, there were lots of activities and best of all, he was free to go outside to an enclosed, secure garden area. Window visits combined with a phone call were also available, but they proved even more heart-breaking than phone conversations. Totem Lodge is located right next to the hospital and the window designated for these visits was close to a pickup and drop off area for service vehicles, and consequently was often noisy, cancelling any chance of John hearing me. After one of these visits, I wrote: *John was overjoyed to see me. Couldn't get enough of looking at me. It was hard, seeing his eyes and being so close. Cut through my heart. We touched hands on either side of the glass. I so hate this! It is like having salt poured on an open wound. I cried all the way home.*

Sometimes, he would wave me to come in and seemed hurt and disappointed when I stayed outside. After the location for these visits was shifted to a window that was lined with a fine wire mesh so it was like looking through the bars of a cage, I refused to take part in them any longer.

I was overjoyed in late July when once-a-week in-person visits were finally permitted, but my relief was short-lived. The visits were conducted outside on a concrete patio where two long garden tables were situated in front of a small fishpond that was backed by ornamental trees. It looked very peaceful, but it was even closer to the noisy service area than the windows of our earlier visits. Now the Health Care Assistant (HCA) supervising the visit met me at the patio gate and, after providing me with a new mask, sanitizing my hands, and asking me the standard COVID questions, she directed me to sit at one end of a six-foot-long table. A moment later she escorted John out to the garden and settled him at the other end of the table, admonishing both of us to remain seated until the visit was over.

John was dressed in a hospital pajama top and jeans that weren't his own, he had a large bruise above his left wrist and scrapes to the back of his hand. He was delighted to see me and kept getting up because he wanted to hug me, but each time the HCA gently guided him back to his chair. I had brought pictures to show him, but was not allowed to give them to him, and they were too small for him to see at a distance, nor could he hear most of the questions I asked. In the end I mostly listened as he voiced his concerns about the traffic on the highway and the trees that needed to be trimmed. For a few moments he was distracted by the birds flitting in and out of the garden, and once he said he would like to go home, but it was a mild statement as if he knew it was not possible. He spent a lot of time removing his glasses and putting them back on. Then for a while we just sat in silence. When it was time to leave, the HCA asked if he wanted to go inside for an ice cream snack. He thought that was okay and left without a backward glance. I, on the other hand, fought tears as I walked back to my car.

The visits improved after I started using the remote microphone that came with John's processor, but it continued to be a challenge to remain six feet apart, especially when it was time to leave because he always wanted to give me a good-bye hug. One day when he persisted in coming towards me, the HCA said sternly, "Rosella, you have to leave!" Not knowing what else to do, I turned away from John's outstretched arms and went out the gate, but as I walked down the drive to my car, I couldn't get his hurt, betrayed expression out of my thoughts. I felt more frustrated, angry, and guilty than I ever have in my life.

I was not alone in my anguish—caregivers all over the province were dealing with the same issue, and it wasn't all about visiting opportunities. Because of COVID and, at least here on the Sunshine Coast, the high cost of housing, care homes were faced with acute staff shortages. Instead of being able to focus on activities for residents, activity coordinators were spending much of their time arranging visiting times, and the rest of the staff were hard pressed to provide basic care. As a result, John often showed up dressed in strange outfits that were not his own, without his processor, and several times sporting more scrapes and bruises that no one could explain. Not being allowed into the facility, I had no idea what his living arrangements were until the HCA kindly sent me a picture of his section of the four-bed ward he was in. I was comforted by the hominess of the space, and especially by the familiar blanket I'd sent from home that was covering his bed, but I was concerned by the lack of privacy for him since only a curtain separated him from the three other occupants of the room.

As other caregivers were doing, I wrote to every agency I could think of to petition for designated caregivers, following the same protocols as staff, to be permitted to help in the care of our loved ones. My letters were received and acknowledged, but the fear of COVID entering the care homes was just too great, and caregivers remained isolated from the care home team.

Recognizing that anger was only making things worse, I focused on making my in-person visits with John be the best they could be with what was available. I found that if I could get the HCA to divert John at the end of the visit with an invitation to come and have a treat or to help with something, he would leave of his own accord and I could slip away unnoticed, comforted by the knowledge that in five minutes he would forget that I'd even been there. One day when he grew restless and got to his feet, I got up with him and, keeping six feet between us, followed him to the fishpond and around the patio, talking about what we saw. The HCA was worried until she saw that I was being very strict about keeping my distance, and for a while it seemed to satisfy John. I discovered, too, that if he had a treat during the visit, he was less likely to get restless.

"Just be present," my therapist said when I asked him how I could make my visits with John more meaningful, but I found this was much easier said than done. I did find that it helped if I focussed on observing what John was doing, rather than on what I wasn't doing, as did accepting the fact that the emotions I was imagining John to be feeling were mine and not his.

"John is not in distress," his doctor said, and overall, I had to agree. There might be moments when he couldn't do what he wanted, but he never asked to come home with me, and when I compared him to the tortured soul he was when he first went into care, I realized how much better off he was in this safe place where the staff were kind and caring and his needs were being met without the anger and resentment he had received from me. There were amusing moments as well. On one visit he was wearing a bib, and when the HCA lifted it to connect the microphone to his processor, I saw a collection of spoons and forks protruding from his pocket. Noticing my curious expression, the HCA laughed and said, "He doesn't like to surrender his cutlery."

One day, John was in the middle of a story and refused to move when our visiting time was over. Another visitor was awaiting her turn, and the HCA was getting desperate. "Do you mind if I call in another resident to help?" she asked me. As I discovered later, John and this lady resident had become quite close—in fact, he sometimes referred to her as his wife.

"Not a problem," I said.

Ellie was a sparse little woman who looked as if she was on an urgent mission as she pushed her walker into the visiting room. Only, instead of going to John as the HCA wanted, she made a beeline for me, and it took some coaxing before she was turned back to the dining room. All the while, John continued telling his story.

"Don't you want to go with Ellie, John?" the HCA asked. "She's going to the dining room."

John barely glanced at the HCA or at Ellie. "Oh, she's always going there," he said.

For the first time a slight edge crept into the HCA's voice. "Please, John, come with me."

At last, having lost whatever fragile thread he'd had to his story, John slowly got to his feet. "Just a minute," he said, pausing to straighten his arthritic knees. The desperate HCA knelt and vigorously massaged them. "There! How's that?"

Somehow she got both John and Ellie headed for the door, but just before he went through, John looked back at me, and I swear there was a twinkle in his eye as he blew me a kiss.

In August, I was invited to participate in a Residential Care Conference via Zoom in which each member of John's care team reviewed his care plan and answered any questions or concerns I might have. The team included his doctor, the nurse in charge of John's care, a pharmacist, the HCA who handled the visiting and recreation activities, and the care home manager. From the doctor, I learned that John had a chronic kidney disease and abnormal blood cells that could develop into cancer. The nurse said he was a "lovely, pleasant man" who had to be monitored closely because he was at risk of falling and because of his tendency to remove his processor and hide it. Since he still occasionally tried to leave the facility, he wore an electronic wander guard. He was very sociable and eager to help the staff and there was no sign of depression or tears. His right knee and left ankle bothered him, but he continued to spend much of the day walking and would frequently go out to the garden. I asked for and was given permission to take him to the dentist but was told there would be no shifting of the touching rules during our in-person visits. Disturbed by this, I asked if it might be less stressful for John if I did not come at all, but the HCA assured me that I made a positive impact on him, and he was always happy when he was told I was coming.

Not long after the conference I received a package of forms that needed to be completed for Totem Lodge, among them an acknowledgement that the care home would not be responsible for the loss of personal items, including dentures, glasses, and hearing aids. I wrote back that John's processor cost over $10,000 to replace, and since I was not permitted to be in the care home, I could not in any way be responsible for its loss and would not sign the form. I received no response to this letter.

In September, as the days grew cooler, in-person visits were moved indoors to a room that could be accessed directly from outside. Long sticks had been placed on the floor to mark the safe-distance boundary (now extended to eight-feet apart) and to keep residents from crossing this line. For John, a stick on the floor had always represented a tripping hazard. Already in a bad mood before the visit began, he immediately became obsessed with the stick, demanding that the HCA remove it. When she refused, he got to his feet and picked it up and for a moment they had a tug-of-war, with him threatening to hit her with it. Finally she wrenched it free, but as one end of the stick swung close to my face, he yelled at her and grabbed for it again. Fortunately she kept it beyond his reach. In an instant he forgot about the stick and reached for me instead, and when the HCA stepped between us to divert him, his anger flared again. Nothing I said calmed him, and clearly disgusted with the whole business, he turned and went back inside to the dining room, leaving me feeling as if I'd failed him once again.

In mid-September, my request to take John for a dental appointment was realized. I was masked when I met him outside the care home door early one morning. He was also masked but gowned as well, and I had generously applied sanitizer not just to my hands but also to the steering wheel and door handles of the car. He was delighted to see me, and when I reached across and squeezed his hand, it felt so right that I almost started to cry.

At the dentist's office, strict COVID protocols were being followed, but I was able to go with him into the examining room so I could help him understand the dental assistant's instructions as she cleaned his teeth. She was horrified by the state of his mouth. His teeth were covered with debris and encrusted with plaque, and his gums were inflamed and bleeding. John was patient during the hour-long cleaning and when it was over, as a reward for both of us, I asked if he'd like to go for a ride. He nodded eagerly, and his eyes were bright as we drove past his old haunts. Since there had been no time specified for his return, I stopped at our home where he was able to go to the washroom and I was able to make him some lunch. No one had visited me there in weeks, and I felt it was a perfectly safe place for him to be. And for the first time in over four months we were able to hug each other.

When I finally brought him back to the care home, I thanked the HCA for this gift then left. This time, the tears I shed on the way home were from joy, not sorrow.

Throughout the fall I was able to take John for more appointments. Some were follow-up visits to the dentist where I discovered that his teeth and gums were much healthier, thanks to the Waterpik I had purchased for him, and the greater care that the staff were taking with his dental hygiene. Two appointments were to the optometrist's offices where I ordered new glasses for him. Each time I took him out, we would go for another long drive and stop at our house for coffee and a treat. On those days we were both happy and close, and when our time was up, we were both ready to return to our new lives—he, because the care home was now the place where he felt safest, and me because as much as I loved the hours with him, I was also exhausted by them.

During this time, to cope with our grief and the heartache of learning to live on our own, Brian and two other caregivers and myself were occasionally meeting for dinner. One caregiver's partner had recently died, and the other's husband had been admitted to the hospital's dementia ward. For a few hours the four of us would enjoy each other's company, talk about our frustrations, and find the humour in some of the tough situations we were facing. I always went home feeling uplifted and stronger.

Brian's wife, Heather, was also in Totem Lodge, but unlike John, she was confined to bed and was not even able to feed herself. Our visiting times were often back-to-back, and we fell into the habit of going for coffee afterwards to commiserate on the frustrations we were encountering. Gradually, we began to realize that we were feeling something much more than just friendship and as the months rolled on it became harder and harder for us to be apart. Finally, with much trepidation on either side, we entered into a relationship that neither of us would ever have considered had our spouses not been in care with absolutely no prospects of ever coming home.

This did not end the anguish we were both feeling as our partners continued to decline. In Heather's case, it was more of a physical decline related to her dementia. As her mobility steadily decreased, she was dependent upon the staff for everything from hygiene to feeding. Worried that staff shortages were limiting the time that HCAs could devote to feeding her, Brian asked to be designated an "essential visitor" so he could come in to feed her at least one meal a day. By sheer persistence he managed to obtain permission to feed her lunch during the week, but it was a tenuous arrangement because the only place he was allowed to be was a room near the in-person visiting area. Heather's bed would be wheeled into this room and her lunch tray brought there. If someone else needed that room, Brian's "essential visit" was cancelled, and he was not permitted to be there on weekends or holidays, or if a meeting was scheduled in the same room.

Soon other caregivers were asking for the same privilege, and to accommodate their needs, Brian's visits were curtailed even more.

He was devastated in the second week of December when he was informed that they were cancelled completely. Five days later it was determined that Heather was "palliative," and consequently Brian could come and go to her room as often as he wanted. By this time, she was almost comatose, and there was nothing he could do except sit by her side and sing to her the love songs they once sang together. Three days later the woman who had shared his life for more than fifty years died. Nothing could ease his grief or the anger he felt towards the health care system that had so failed them both.

That same month while John was being treated for a severe urinary tract infection, tests showed that he had a cancerous tumour in his bladder, which in accordance with his advance health directive would not be removed. His behaviour was also causing concern, with an escalation of violent incidents, usually when he was being deterred from "looking after" the other residents, who were not at all happy with his interference in their routines. In January 2021 after he severely bruised the arm of the HCA who was trying to distract him, he was put on an "Urgent" transfer list for a secure ward. Since the only two secure wards on the Sunshine Coast were already full, his anger issues were treated with increased medications. These made him so groggy that on one visit to the dentist he could not understand how to sit in the chair.

It was March before a bed became available at Shorncliffe. Following instructions from the long-term care manager, I collected John and all of his possessions from Totem. He had a dental appointment that day, and when it was over, I brought him home and we sat in front of the fire and held hands. After a short drive along the waterfront, I delivered him to Shorncliffe.

Located at the top of a hill and overlooking the Sechelt waterfront bordering Trail Bay and beyond to the Strait of Georgia, Shornecliffe is a three-level facility with accessible garden areas on the two upper levels. I was delighted that I was able to accompany John to the third- floor ward and though he was very confused, he seemed to like the bright, private room that had been assigned to him. It had a window facing out past some shrubs and a bit of a lawn, and if he stood at a certain angle, he could see the waters of Trail Bay. The room was equipped with an easy chair, a single bed, a bedside table, closets, drawers, and a large ensuite bathroom. I put away the things we'd brought with us and, since I would now be able to have scheduled visits with him in this room, made note of what I could bring to make it even homier.

The HCA on duty had worked in the Adult Day Care program and remembered John well. Because he would have to isolate for fourteen days, she brought dinner to his room. By the time he finished eating, he was so tired that he went to bed and was almost asleep when I quietly slipped away.

Before John's transfer to Shorncliffe, I had requested and been granted permission to take him for weekly drives. In time, these were extended to twice a week with an in-room visit in-between, and for the first time since he was admitted to care, I felt as if I could make a positive difference in his life. As always, he loved the drives, and we happily explored both oceanside routes and wilderness backroads, some that he'd once driven on his own and others that were new to both of us. On one journey, as we passed a familiar landmark, he said in his jumbled way that he'd been there before when he wasn't residing at the "fuzzy-doos." We always topped off our excursions by stopping at our house for coffee and a treat.

He tried to walk in the yard, I wrote after one of our outings, *but his knee hurt, and he was too wobbly. He didn't make a fuss when I took him back to Shorncliffe, but I sensed his sadness. I am always over-whelmed with grief and anger and helplessness when I leave. While my intellect knows I am doing the best thing I can do for him, my emotions have another opinion. Eventually that anger recedes, and I can just love him, but with the loving comes despair.*

Sometimes John's memory was surprisingly acute, and he would point out the turnoff to our road and say, "This is where I used to live. I've walked this many times."

On April 27, 2021, the anniversary of the day he first went into care, I found John in the dining area. He was seated at a table with two women, and they seemed to be enjoying each other's company so much that it took a few moments for him to agree to come with me. This time, I drove along a backroad near Trout Lake, north of Sechelt. I didn't know where we were going, but we were both happy because it was very much like the backroads we used to explore at Clowhom Falls. At one point, I stopped the car and we waited as a grouse slowly made its way across the road. John watched the bird's every move. Later, we drove to the beach at Coopers Green in Halfmoon Bay and he sat on a bench for a while. It was so cold that, even with blankets around him, he didn't want to stay long, but he told me as we drove along Redrooffs Road that he was very familiar with this part of Oregon. Back at Shorncliffe, I went with him to the ward. It was a perfect day until I went to leave, and he wanted to come with me. There was no staff member around, so I took him to the TV area, and he grudgingly sat with some other residents.

You gave him a happy day, I told myself firmly as I walked away, but that didn't ease the sadness I was feeling.

Although I was now permitted to go into John's room, I was still not allowed anywhere else on the ward, a rule I sometimes ignored when I had to leave and could not find any staff member to help make this transition easier. Once, when I'd noticed blood in his urine, I tried to find someone to tell, but no staff was in sight, and finally had to relay the information to the receptionist in the lobby.

I had been assured when John was slated for the secure ward that it would mean he would receive more one-on-one care, but I wasn't convinced this was happening. Certainly, there were legitimate reasons for the absence of staff—often they were looking after a patient in a closed room—but it was worrisome, especially after I visited the garden area one day and saw the uneven paving stones that were a potential hazard for patients with mobility issues.

There were also problems with John's processor. On one occasion I arrived to take him for a drive and found that he had neither glasses nor processor. I tracked down a nurse who said it was locked in a cupboard in the nurse's station because John kept hiding it.

"But without it, he is completely deaf," I protested, wondering how much of the day John was spending without his hearing.

The nurse rolled her eyes. "He has dementia," she said, as if talking to a child. "We have to do what keeps them safe."

Two weeks later I found John sleeping, and although he was wearing his processor, he did not have the controller that was required for it to work. The nurse in charge was the same one who had locked his processor in the nurses' station.

"He keeps hiding it, and we have to look for it!" she exclaimed, obviously forgetting our first conversation.

"Yes," I said, my tongue firmly lodged in my cheek, "he has dementia."

We searched his room, and I found the controller in the pocket of some pants hanging in the bathroom. I wondered why no one had checked the pants when they helped him settle for the night, and if the processor had even been put on the charger.

One day in early May, as I entered the ward for an in-room visit, John came toward me, and his expression was one of relief—as if I had just saved him. He was not happy, but he could not tell me why, and our visit did not go well. He wasn't interested in the book of sea life that we usually looked at together nor in any discussions about our life at Clowhom. He didn't want to be confined to his room and finally headed for the dining area. I said if he went out there, I couldn't go with him, but it didn't matter—he wasn't staying in his room. "I'm done with this," he said crossly.

"Do you want me to come tomorrow?" I asked.

"No," he snapped. "I'm done."

As he made his way to the TV corner, I let myself out, feeling sad and guilty but trying to remind myself that some days he was not going to be happy and that's just the way it was.

I was reassured the following day when we went for another drive, and he was back to his amiable self. We stopped at home for coffee and donuts and then went to a park and sat on a bench and looked at the water. When I drove him back to Shorncliffe, he knew the way up the hill and told me where to turn off. This time, he went inside willingly and was content to sit in the TV area with some of the other residents, allowing me a peaceful exit.

Late the following afternoon an HCA from Shorncliffe called to say that John had fallen and was complaining that his groin was hurting so they were sending him by ambulance to the hospital. She didn't sound concerned and assured me they would call me from the hospital when they had determined what was wrong. Only the hospital didn't call, and when I called them, they said John hadn't arrived. My repeated calls to Shorncliffe to find out what was happening went unanswered. Finally, at eleven thirty that night I got through to the hospital once again and was told that John was being admitted overnight while they determined the extent of his injuries, and if there was anything seriously wrong, they would call me.

I slept little that night, and at six the next morning I called the hospital. The nurse in charge said John had a fractured hip and was awaiting assessment from the orthopedic surgeon. She assured me John was resting and that he was comfortable and calm. Two hours later the doctor called and confirmed that John had a fractured hip, but he also had a brain bleed. Given how this would affect the quality of his life and because of the advance health directive he'd signed, it had been decided that he would be transferred back to Shorncliffe and kept comfortable, but nothing would be done. It was possible, the doctor said, that the bleed would clear up on its own and the fracture, because it was not displaced, would heal in five months.

I arrived at Shorncliffe just after John was returned and to my horror found he was not "comfortable" in any way. He was in severe pain, his arm was badly bruised, and he seemed afraid and vulnerable as he gripped my hand and looked at me so gratefully that it took every bit of will I possessed not to cry. Only when the morphine and sedatives he'd been given finally kicked in and he slept, did I allow my tears to flow.

A nurse came in while John slept and told me that because he was now designated palliative, I could come and go at any hour and stay as long as I wanted. I could also have other visitors in the room at the same time. This was a relief as my sister, Vera, was able to join me in my vigil as I watched him slowly lose his hold on this world that he so did not want to leave. Most of the time he was asleep, waking only when the pain medication wore off and then being in distress until more medication was administered. I held his hand, sponged his face and brow, and sang to him…and thought of our life together, the good times we had shared, walking to the lake, fishing, coaxing a big ling or red snapper to the surface, driving up into the mountains looking for deer, standing on top of the world, looking down at our paradise while a cold breeze washed our cheeks . . .

During the day, staff members from Totem and Shorncliffe dropped by to say goodbye, many of them with tears in their eyes. Even though he could not hear them, they would speak gently to him, offering cheer and caring, and then doing the same for me. It was a reminder that even when things are at their worst, there is still much good in this world.

When John died, I was alone in the room. I was holding his hand and whispering that I loved him, and as his final breath eased from his lips, so it seemed did the pain and the struggle of the last twelve years. He had stopped at last and was at peace.

PERPETUITY

You are with me when the dawn's gentle light
Eases the darkness from the night.
In the joyous trilling of birds in spring
I hear your spirit sing;
In the warmth of lazy summer days
I am reminded of your special ways.
I see you smiling when fall winds so soft
Waft chariots of golden leaves aloft.
Your love that warmed and eased cold winter's chill
Is with me still;
And in the splendour of the sunset's hue,
I am assured that peace has come to you.

Moving On

REFLECTIONS

Our worth is oft reflected in the gaze
Of those who know us better than ourselves,
Until dementia wipes away that truth,
By shattering the mirror in their eyes
That kept our paths aligned with who we are.
And while their image lingers still in ours,
It's soon distorted by their endless needs,
And their reality that has no "us."

Then comes a day, although it breaks our hearts,
When we relinquish them to long term care,
(Or death slips in and steals them away.)
It's then we realize how far we've strayed
From who we were before we made this trek,
And we must take our lives up once again,
Without a compass, or *raison d'être*,
Nor image of the self we used to be.

That's where I was when I met you, my love,
A lonely soul who couldn't find her way,
A stranger in a land that I knew not.
Until one night we dared a sweet embrace
That brought us closer than we could believe,
And in the mirror of your loving gaze
I saw, reflected back, the me I'd lost.
'Twas then I knew the world was mine again.

John's death was not the end of my caregiving journey. For a while, I was in shock, partly because I could not believe this dear man who had been such a vital part of my life was gone and partly because it was hard to grasp that the responsibility for his care was gone from my shoulders.

But grief, like joy, cannot sustain itself, and gradually my sorrow eased, and I began the transition to life without him. The first step in this process was selling the home we had shared. The property was too big for me to manage alone and held too many memories that were better left in the past. Once it was sold, I faced dismantling and finding new homes for the mountain of bits and pieces that had accumulated in the thirty-seven years we had spent together. Eventually, with the help of Brian and my family and friends, the final load was carted away, and as I drove down the drive for the last time, I felt both sadness and a lightness of spirit that had been missing for many years.

As with the end of most journeys, however, there was a time now for reflection, for looking back at all that had transpired since the day the doctor confirmed that John had dementia. I was reminded then of Kathy Thomas asking us caregivers what we had gained from our caregiver experience. It had seemed a strange question at the time, but now I realized that as much as caregiving had taken from me, it had also enhanced my life. It had enabled me to recognize strengths I never knew I had and to witness the generosity and caring of people, including strangers. I had learned to leave my debt ledger behind when I reached out and asked for help, and slowly I came to accept that the negative emotions I had experienced were not just involuntary, they were also warnings from my subconscious to tell me that I had to make changes if I wanted to maintain my health so I could continue to be John's advocate. Instead of dismissing or judging them, I had gradually discovered strategies to cope with my feelings of anger, fear, disappointment, and guilt—strategies that can be applied to many situations other than caregiving. I came to accept that just as I had not caused, could not cure, and could not control John's disease, neither could I cause, cure or control other life events, including COVID, climatic disasters and love.

I learned, too, that many more resources are needed to help persons with dementia and their caregivers. Care homes need to include caregivers and volunteers as an essential part of the team, taking advantage of and valuing the support they can give, enabling them to continue—following the same safety protocols as regular staff members—to provide that support even when there is a pandemic or a virus in the community. And because it reduces the high cost of building and maintaining care homes as well as the emotional upheaval that going into care causes to persons with dementia and their caregivers, health authorities need to provide more supports for those caring for persons with dementia at home. Flexible day programs that address the individual needs of persons with dementia and are available seven days a week and on holidays will give caregivers time to re-energize and focus on their own needs. Affordable and flexible home care opportunities that meet the needs of both the caregiver and the person with dementia will reduce caregiver stress, enabling them to provide care longer. More counselling services and better communication avenues to enable caregivers to reach out and find help when they need it as well as increased financial support for community organizations dedicated to supporting caregivers are vital to maintaining their equilibrium. These may seem to be utopian demands, but they are very doable and much less costly than the current system.

The journey of caregiving someone with dementia is not unlike experiencing a war. Instead of facing a hostile nation or citizen rebellion, a caregiver deals with a disease that presses forward despite medications and therapies, its weapons being the emotional and physical deterioration of both the caregiver and the person with dementia. And just as in any conflict, a bonding happens among those who are fighting on the same side of the war, and deep connections are formed that continue long after the caregiving journey has ended.

We can never know what the next day holds for us. In the midst of my despair, I could not have believed it possible that there would still be a meaningful future waiting for me when I was no longer a caregiver, or that I might find love again.

I will always miss John, as Brian will always miss Heather. They are a big part of each of us and always will be. We are comforted now by knowing that we were present for them right until the end, doing the best we could to help them in their journey, letting them know they were dearly loved, and that is as much as any human can ask of another.

And today, as I walk along a wooded trail, my hand tucked into Brian's, I feel the wind softly brushing my cheeks with promise.

AFTERMATH

Smoky sky and soft swell,
Four loons swimming,
And me paddling forth.
Hard pull on the right,
Soft pull on the left,
Bow straight as it slides
Between islets.

Mergansers stop to preen
On rocky shore,
And I pause to watch,
Gently swayed by the surf.
Mustering courage,
I turn my kayak
And face the waves.

Handle gripped and blade dipped,
Bow cresting wave,
Hull skimming the top,
And bridging the trough.
Blissful harmony—
The kayak, the sky,
The sea and me.

APPENDIX I

Selected Resource List For Caregivers

Note: I do not endorse any of these sites. I have simply conducted a Google search of caregiver services available and selected those that I deemed worthy of further exploration. Sites may not be secure.

CANADA FEDERAL

Alzheimer Society of Canada
https://alzheimer.ca/

Alzheimer's Association
Similar to the Alzheimer Society of Canada, this organization's website provides free resources for all those who are touched by dementia.
https://www.alz.org/ca

However, specific for caregivers is the Caregiver Center. https://www.alz.org/help-support/caregiving

ALZLIVE
Digital lifestyle and news platform for family caregivers of
Alzheimer's and dementia patients in US and Canada. Owned by
Kelso Publishing Inc.
https://alzlive.com/

Comfort Keepers Canada
Caregiver Resources (Private)
https://www.comfortkeepers.ca/caregiver-resources/

Comfort Life
Web Resources for Families (Private)
https://seniorcommunity.org/

Dementia Connections
Canadian magazine featuring inspiring stories, expert advice, and
the latest developments in dementia care and research.
https://dementiaconnections.ca/

Dementia Friendly Communities
https://www.dementiafriendlyalberta.ca/resources/useful-
information.html

Dunn & Bradstreet
Listing and details of Home Health Care Services Companies
in Canada
https://www.dnb.com/business-directory/company-information.
home_health_care_services.ca.html

Government Assistance and Funding for Caregivers in Canada
https://elizz.com/planning/
government-assistance-and-funding-for-caregivers-in-canada/

EmentalHealth Services – Find Mental Health Services in your area.
A non-profit initiative of the Children's Hospital of Eastern Ontario (CHEO) dedicated to improving the mental health of children, youth and families. Links to services across Canada.
https://www.ementalhealth.ca/

Forward with dementia: A guide to living with dementia. (A dementia partnership program registered in Australia, Canada, Netherlands, Poland and the United Kingdom)
https://www.forwardwithdementia.org/

Government of Canada Veterans' Affairs Caregiver Zone
https://www.veterans.gc.ca/eng/family-caregiver/housing-and-home-life/caregiver-zone

Government of Canada Dementia Overview
https://www.canada.ca/en/public-health/services/diseases/dementia.html

Government of Canada Benefits for Caregivers
https://www.canada.ca/en/financial-consumer-agency/services/caring-someone-ill/benefits-tax-credits-caregivers.html

Legal Line: Access to Canadian Laws – caregiver benefits
https://www.legalline.ca/legal-answers/caregiver-benefits/

Morning Star Lodge: An Indigenous Community-Based Health Research Lab
https://www.indigenoushealthlab.com/

Dementia Caregiver Toolkit
https://static1.squarespace.com/
static/566604882399a3d028922f9a/t/5fa5a5f7a0c5116b30c5
1ac9/1604691448331/links.pdf

Provincial Caregiving Resources List
https://healthexperiences.ca/family-caregiving/
provincial-caregiving-organizations-resources

Teva Canada (Private)
https://www.tevacanada.com/en/canada/support-for-caregivers/

211— Canada's primary source of information for government
and community-based, non-clinical health and social services.
https://211.ca/

Victorian Order of Nurses for Canada Respite Services in Nova
Scotia and Ontario
https://www.von.ca/

CANADA PROVINCIAL

Alberta

Alberta Health Services. Dementia Advice provides support
for people living with dementia and their caregivers, including
tele-triage, health advice, and available resources.
https://www.albertahealthservices.ca/main/search/Pages/Search.
aspx?k=Dementia

Alzheimer Society Calgary Caregiver Support Group
https://www.alzheimercalgary.ca/find-support/support-groups

Bridge to Care Specialized Care for all Life Stages and Abilities
https://www.bridgetocare.org/

Caregivers of Alberta Resources and Support
https://www.caregiversalberta.ca/

Covenant Health Resources and Supports for Caregivers in
Alberta Last updated 2018
https://seniorsnetworkcovenant.ca/wp-content/uploads/
Inventory-of-Resources-and-Supports-for-Caregivers-in-Alberta-
Dementia-Supports.pdf

Dementia Friendly Communities
https://www.dementiafriendlyalberta.ca/resources/useful-
information.html

Inform Alberta Province Wide Service Directory for Caregivers
https://informalberta.ca/public/results/relatedSubjects.
do?taxonomyQueryId=5585

British Columbia

Family Caregivers of British Columbia
https://www.familycaregiversbc.ca/

Government of British Columbia Caring for Seniors
https://www2.gov.bc.ca/gov/content/family-social-supports/
seniors/caring-for-seniors
https://www2.gov.bc.ca/gov/content/family-social-supports/
seniors/caring-for-seniors/caring-for-the-caregiver

HealthLinkBC Dementia Support for Caregivers
https://www.healthlinkbc.ca/illnesses-conditions/dementia/
dementia-support-caregivers

Island Health Dementia Caregiver Services
https://www.islandhealth.ca/learn-about-health/seniors/dementia

March of Dimes Canada Caregiver Resources
https://www.marchofdimes.ca/en-ca/aboutus/landr/Pages/
Resources-Caregiver.aspx

VGH UBC Hospital Foundation Caregivers Clinic
https://vghfoundation.ca/brain-dementia-caregivers-clinic/

Vancouver Coastal Health Caregiver Support Services
http://www.vch.ca/your-care/home-community-care/
care-options/caregiver-support

Manitoba

Alzheimer Society of Manitoba
https://alzheimer.mb.ca/we-can-help/resources/

Government of Manitoba Resources for Caregivers
https://www.gov.mb.ca/seniors/docs/caregiver_inventory.pdf

Newfoundland

Alzheimer Society of Newfoundland and Labrador
https://alzheimer.ca/nl/en/help-support/
find-support-newfoundland-labrador

Caregivers Newfoundland Resource Links
https://www.caregiversnl.com/resources/

Government of Newfoundland and Labrador Provincial Home
Support Program
https://www.gov.nl.ca/hcs/files/personsdisabilities-pdf-home-
support-program-client-handbook.pdf

New Brunswick

Alzheimer Society of New Brunswick
First Link and other Social Supports
https://socialsupportsnb.ca/en/program/first-link

Forward With Dementia
Provincial Resources to Support Persons Living with Dementia
and Their Care Partners – New Brunswick
https://www.forwardwithdementia.org/ca-en/wp-content/
uploads/sites/7/2021/07/Provincial-Resources_NB_FWD_EN_
PDF.pdf

Government of New Brunswick Caregivers Guide
https://www2.gnb.ca/content/dam/gnb/Departments/sd-ds/pdf/
Seniors/CaregiversGuide.pdf

New Brunswick Home Support Association
Links and Resources
http://nbhsa.ca/english/links-resources

Social Supports New Brunswick, Department of Health
Dementia
https://socialsupportsnb.ca/en/simple_page/dementia

Rosella M. Leslie

Saint Andrews Dementia Caregiving Guide
https://www.townofsaintandrews.ca/wp-content/uploads/2021/06/Dementia-Caregiving-Guide-2021.pdf

Northwest Territories

Alzheimer Society of Alberta and Northwest Territories
https://alzheimer.ca/ab/en

Avens, Yellowknife, NWT Resource List
https://www.avensseniors.com/resources/useful-resources

Government of Northwest Territories – NWT Caregivers' Guide
https://www.hss.gov.nt.ca/sites/hss/files/nwt-caregivers-guide.pdf

Inuvialuit Regional Corporation Dementia Awareness
and Intervention
https://irc.inuvialuit.com/service/health-and-wellness

Nova Scotia

Alzheimer Society of Nova Scotia
https://alzheimer.ca/ns/en

Caregivers Nova Scotia Resources for friends and family
giving care
https://caregiversns.org/
https://caregiversns.org/how-we-help/peer-support-groups/other-support-groups/

811 Nova Scotia Caring for a Relative Who Has Dementia
https://811.novascotia.ca/health_topics/
caring-for-a-relative-who-has-dementia/

Government of Nova Scotia Home Care Resources
https://novascotia.ca/dhw/ccs/home-care.asp

Nova Scotia Health Respite and Caregiver Support
https://www.nshealth.ca/content/respite-and-caregiver-support

Pictou-Antigonish Regional Library List of Dementia Resources
http://www.parl.ns.ca/projects/healthroom/alzheimers.php

Nunavut

The Government of Nunavut Home and Continuing Care
https://www.gov.nu.ca/health/information/
home-and-continuing-care

Ontario

Acclaim Health Caregiver Support
https://acclaimhealth.ca/programs/dementia-care/
caregiver-support-groups/

Alzheimer Society, Toronto
https://alz.to/

Baycrest
https://Baycrest.org/
https://www.baycrest.org/Baycrest/Education-Training/
Educational-Resources/Dementia-Resources-Around-
The-World/Dementia-Resources-for-Patients/
Support-Programs

Canadian Mental Health Association
https://cmha.ca/
https://cmha.bc.ca/documents/alzheimers-disease-2/

Canadian Red Cross – Home Care Services
https://www.redcross.ca/how-we-help/
community-health-services-in-canada/home-care-services

Caregiver Exchange Service Listings
https://www.caregiverexchange.ca/

Caregiver Support Services, Mount Sinai Hospital
https://www.mountsinai.on.ca/care/psych/patient-programs/
geriatric-psychiatry/prc-dementia-resources-for-primary-care/
community-resources-and-directories
https://www.circleofcare.com/

Dementia Carers -- Provides free of charge clinical services and
group programs for care partners of a person living with dementia at partner locations across Ontario.
https://www.dementiacarers.ca/care-partner-programs/

The Dementia Society Ottawa and Renfrew Counties
https://dementiahelp.ca/

Government of Ontario Caregiving Guide
https://www.ontario.ca/document/
guide-programs-and-services-seniors/caregiving

Home and Community Care Support Services
http://healthcareathome.ca/ww/en/Getting-Care/
Patient-and-Caregiver-Resources/Helpful-Links

Lakehead University Centre for Education and Research on
Aging and Health
Links to Resources for People Living with Dementia
https://cerah.lakeheadu.ca/

McGill/Steinberg Centre for Simulation and Interactive Learning
https://www.mcgill.ca/medsimcentre/community-outreach/
dementia/dementia-resources
https://www.mcgill.ca/medsimcentre/community-outreach/
dementia/dementia-your-companion-guide

The Ontario Caregiver Organization Support for Caregivers
https://ontariocaregiver.ca/for-caregivers/

Helpline: 1-833-416-2273 (CARE). Phone and Live Chat.
Ontario Caregiver Coalition
https://www.ontariocaregivercoalition.ca/resources

University of Toronto Family Care Office
https://familycare.utoronto.ca/eldercare/caregiver-support/

VHA Home Healthcare Non-profit organization offering health
care and support services
https://www.vha.ca/dementia-care/heart-in-mind/

Prince Edward Island

Adult Day Programs
https://www.princeedwardisland.ca/en/information/health-pei/
adult-day-programs

Alzheimer Society of Prince Edward Island
https://alzheimer.ca/pei/en

Forward With Dementia Provincial Resources to Support Persons
with Dementia and Care Partners
https://www.forwardwithdementia.org/
ca-en/wp-content/uploads/sites/7/2021/10/
Provincial-Resources_PEI_FWD_EN.pdf

Health PEI
https://www.princeedwardisland.ca/en/information/health-pei/
seniors-mental-health-resource-teams

HOSPICE PEI Caregiver Support Resources
https://hospicepei.ca/caregiver-support-resources/

Quebec

Alzheimer Society of Montreal
https://alzheimermontreal.ca/

AmiQuebec Includes Services for Caregivers – Non-profit
https://amiquebec.org/

Appui Proches Audents Resources for Caregivers
https://www.lappui.org/en/

Government of Quebec Services for Seniors
https://www.quebec.ca/en/family-and-support-for-individuals/
seniors
https://ciusss-ouestmtl.gouv.qc.ca/en/care-services/
west-island-territory/services-for-seniors-and-
people-with-decreasing-independence/
services-for-seniors-and-people-with-decreasing-independence/

Hope For Dementia Advocacy Group
https://hopefordementia.org/

Resource List of Mental Health Services, Quebec
https://www.ementalhealth.ca/Quebec/Dementia-including-
Alzheimers/index.php?m=heading&ID=110

Santé Montérégie Portal Home Care for People with Loss
of Autonomy
https://www.santemonteregie.qc.ca/en/services/home-support/
home-care-people-loss-autonomy

Saskatchewan

Alzheimer Society of Saskatchewan
https://alzheimer.ca/sk/en

Dementia Supports in Rural Saskatchewan
https://www.ruraldementiask.ca/

Government of Saskatchewan Dementia Services and Support
https://www.saskatchewan.ca/residents/health/
diseases-and-conditions/dementia

Rosella M. Leslie

Saskatchewan Health Authority
https://www.saskhealthauthority.ca/your-health/conditions-
diseases-services/healthline-online/uf4984
https://www.saskatoonhealthregion.ca/locations_services/
Services/Senior-Health/Pages/North-Saskatchewan-Dementia-
Assessment-Unit.aspx

Saskatoon Council on Aging Caregiver Information and Support
http://www.saskatooncaregiver.ca/resources.html

University of Saskatchewan Rural and Remote Memory Clinic
https://cchsa-ccssma.usask.ca/ruraldementiacare/Rural%20
Remote%20Memory%20Clinic.php#ObjectivesandGoals

Yukon

Government of Yukon Resources for Caregivers
https://yukon.ca/en/health-and-wellness/care-services/find-
resources-caregivers
https://yukon.ca/en/caregiver-support-group

Yukon Division Canadian Mental Health Association
https://yukon.cmha.ca/home/mental-health/
learn-about-mental-health/alzheimers-disease/

Yukon Seniors and Elders Alzheimer's Articles
https://yukon-seniors-and-elders.org/index.php/
ga-home/132-alzheimer-s

Links To Selected Ted Talks And Online Videos

"The Power of Vulnerability" Brené Brown https://www.ted.com/talks/brene_brown_the_power_of_vulnerability?language=en

"Compassion Fatigue in Caregiving" Patricia
Smith, TEDxSanJuanIsland
https://www.youtube.com/watch?v=7keppA8XRas

Dr. Wayne Dyer (1940–2015) Inspirational books and videos on self-development and spiritual growth
https://www.drwaynedyer.com/

Escape the Custard—A New Plan for Anxious Feelings Neil
Hughes, TEDxLeamingtonSpa
https://www.walkingoncustard.com/anxious/
https://enhughesiasm.com/anxiety

Teepa Snow Positive Approach to Care Articles and videos on dementia care
https://teepasnow.com/

"Self-care for Caregivers" Linda Ercoli, TEDxUCLA
https://www.youtube.com/watch?v=H3RQ9-hOuIE

"The Space Between Self-Esteem and Self-Compassion"
Dr. Kristin Neff, TEDxCentennialParkWomen
https://www.youtube.com/watch?v=IvtZBUSplr4
https://self-compassion.org/

"Three Secrets of Resilient People" Dr. Lucy
Hone, TEDxChristchurch
https://www.youtube.com/watch?v=NWH8N-BvhAw

Endorsements

Reading Rosella Leslie's *Losing Us—A Dementia Caregiver's Journey* is like having an understanding and helpful friend at your side on the journey of caring for someone with dementia, sharing her toolbox full of essentials like validation, inspiration, strength, comfort, understanding, and humour along with helpful tips she learned along the way in her own caregiving experience.

I wish I could have read *Losing Us* when I was at an earlier stage of this journey. I think it would have helped me be kinder with my mother *and* myself along the way. In sharing her story Rosella has essentially also written mine, validating the immensity of the roller coaster ride of being a caregiver to a beloved family member with dementia while making sure to point out the strength it brings out in us, as well as showing us the path to mitigating the emotional toll it takes.

And, oh…her poems…they touch that vulnerable pulse of our experience so perfectly!

This book is also a treatise on what is needed by that proverbial "village" to honourably care for the people afflicted with this disease as well as supporting the families who care for them.

Thank you so much, Rosella, for having the courage to share such an unvarnished and real account of your experiences. With *Losing Us* you have given us all a gift.

Anna Wright, Caregiver, May 1, 2022.

I first met Rosella Leslie at the Senior Adult Mental Health offices where the Caregiver Support Group was meeting. It was February 2018, shortly after I had moved to the Sunshine Coast with my late wife Lyn, and at that meeting I listened to Rosella's heartfelt out-pouring of grief and anger over the course her husband's dementia was following and the toll it was taking on her and her relationship.

Although my experiences with my wife's dementia were different than Rosella's, as every case is different, the devastating effects the disease has on the patient are well known. What is not so well known is the horrible, brutal, soul-crushing effects it has on a devoted spouse who is struggling to do the jobs of a team of trained medical professionals, testing their resolve, sanity and even humanity twenty-four hours a day, in the mistaken belief that it is their duty to carry on until they drop.

When Rosella asked me to read *Losing Us – A Dementia Caregiver's Journey*, I was first honoured and then very hesitant. I was hon-oured first to be trusted with the unpublished manuscript but once I started reading, it was so brutally honest that it brought back all the memories that time was finally allowing to fade from my own time as a caregiver. She hides nothing in the writing of *Losing Us*. She lays her heart and soul on the table for all to see as she takes the reader through all the stages of the journey that she and John were forced to endure. Having been present at the Caregiver Group meetings, I can attest to the accuracy and honesty of Rosella's depiction of events as she describes them because I remember a lot of the situations that she talked about there.

Not a book for the faint of heart, *Losing Us* can almost be consid-ered a road map for caregivers who are just starting the journey. While her memoir might describe situations that not every care-giver will come up against, Rosella gives the reader a very good idea of what could happen on any dementia journey if someone is unfortunate enough to be directed down that path.

I truly hope Mother Nature allows science to find a cure for this horrible, demoralizing, dehumanizing disease.

Mark Garland (Retired Caregiver), May 4, 2022

Citations

1 Mayo Clinic Staff, "Stress relief from laughter? It's no joke," Mayo Clinic, July 29, 2021, https://www.mayoclinic.org/healthy-lifestyle/stress-management/in-depth/stress-relief/art-20044456.

2 Marilyn A. Mendoza, "The Healing Power of Laughter in Death and Grief: Humor in Hospice," *Psychology Today*, Nov 7, 2016, , https://www.psychologytoday.com/ca/blog/understanding-grief/201611/the-healing-power-laughter-in-death-and-grief.

3 Judy Croon, "The Superpower of Humour," TEDxStMaryCSSchool, May 31, 2018, video, 16:04, https://www.youtube.com/watch?v=_oFQLllk_LM.

4 Jennifer Aaker and Naomi Bagdonas, "Why Great Leaders Take Humour Seriously," TedMonterey, July 2021, video, 9:10, https://www.ted.com/talks/jennifer_aaker_and_naomi_bagdonas_why_great_leaders_take_humor_seriously

5 Amy Lyle, "Finding the Funny in Crummy," TEDxBeaconStreet, Jan 11, 2021, video, 9:09, https://www.youtube.com/watch?v=nVl7tEZ6p04.

6 "Minds in Motion," Alzheimer Society of BC, accessed January 22, 2022, https://alzheimer.ca/bc/en/help-support/programs-services/minds-motion.

7 "Logotherapy," Wikipedia, accessed August 23, 2021, https://en.wikipedia.org/wiki/Logotherapy

8 Viktor E. Frankl, *Man's Search for Meaning*, June 1, 2005, Beacon Press; First published 1946, page 133.

9 Julie Sternberg and Eve Yohalem, hosts, "Edith Eger: "I Go Through the Valley of the Shadow of Death. I Don't Camp There," Book Dreams (podcast), May 6, 2021, accessed August 24, 2021, https://lithub.com/edith-eger-i-go-through-the-valley-of-the-shadow-of-death-i-dont-camp-there/.

10 Edith Eva Eger, *The Choice: Embrace the Possible* (New York: Scribner, 2018), page 237

11 Neil Hughes, "A new plan for anxious feelings: escape the custard!" TEDxLeamingtonSpa, March 29, 2016, video, 14:14, https://www.youtube.com/watch?v=bM06o26PCDQ&ab_channel=TEDxTalks.

12 Lucy Hone, "The three secrets of resilient people," TEDxChristchurch, August 2019, video, 16:21, https://www.ted.com/talks/lucy_hone_the_three_secrets_of_resilient_people.

13 "I'm caring for a person living with dementia," Alzheimer Society, https://alzheimer.ca/en/help-support/im-caring-person-living-dementia.

14 Teepa Snow, "Positive Approach to Care," *www.teepasnow.com*, accessed August 25, 2021.

15 Manuel J. Smith, *When I Say No, I Feel Guilty,* (New York: Bantam Books, 1975) page 4

16 Kristin Neff, "The Difference Between Self Compassion and Self Esteem," TEDx Centennial Park Women, Feb 6, 2013, video, 19:00, https://self-compassion.org/.

17 Kristin Neff, "Self-Compassion," https://self-compassion.
org/. Kristin Neff is Co-Founder of the Center for
Mindful Self-Compassion.

18 Amelia Gillies, Support and Education Coordinator,
Alzheimer Society of B.C. Email November 5, 2021.

19 "Deaths from COVID-19 have disproportionately affected
seniors living in long-term care. Although only 1% of
Canadians reside in long-term care, deaths in these facilities
represent 80% of all COVID deaths in Canada." Maria Chung,
"COVID-19 and long-term care," *BC Medical Journal*, vol.
62, no. 6, (July August 2020): 206, https://bcmj.org/
cohp-covid-19/covid-19-and-long-term-care.

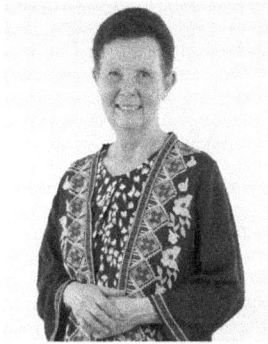

About the Author

Rosella M. Leslie is the author of The *Cougar Lady: Legendary Trapper of Sechelt Inlet, The Federov Legacy, Drift Child* and *The Goat Lady's Daughter*. She has co-authored *Stain Upon the Sea: West Coast Salmon Farming, Bright Seas, Pioneer Spirits: The History of the Sunshine Coast, Updated and Revised* and *Sea Silver: Inside British Columbia's Salmon-Farming Industry*. Her awards for her excellence in writing include winner of the Federation of BC Writer's Best of BC Writing Competition (1986), co-winner of third prize for the BC Historical Writing Competition (1997); co-winner of the Roderick Haig-Brown Regional Prize (2004); and honourable mention in *Prairie Fire's* 2016 fiction contest.

A founding member of the Sunshine Coast Festival of the Written Arts, Rosella is a member of The Writers' Union and a leader of the Memory Café in Sechelt. You can connect with her through her websites www.rosellaleslie.com and www.quintessentialwriters.com.

When she's not writing, you can find Rosella hiking, running, and gardening in Halfmoon Bay, BC with Brian and his beautiful golden retriever, Gracie.

CPSIA information can be obtained
at www.ICGtesting.com
Printed in the USA
BVHW040544180523
664268BV00019B/35